Overcoming Overeating—
a whole-person approach to weight loss

"A comprehensive remedy for weight loss. Lisa rightly views weight problems as having their origin in not just physical, but also mental, emotional, and spiritual arenas…An invaluable resource to the countless people struggling in this area of their life."

—David Hawkins, PhD, psychologist, director of the Marriage Recovery Center, and author of *When Pleasing Others Is Hurting You*

"A practical, sustainable, and results-oriented approach that will guide you to permanent mind change…*Overcoming Overeating* provides both the why and the how toward becoming the new, healthy you."

—J. Ron Eaker, MD, physician and author of *Fat-Proof Your Family* and *A Woman's Guide to Hormone Health*

"If you have struggled with overeating, this resource will provide you with practical help. Lisa walks with you through the book…giving you a clear strategy to restore balance to your life in the area of eating. I highly recommend this work."

—Scott Forsmith, LCSW-R

What Health-Care Experts Are Saying About Other Books by Lisa Morrone, PT

Overcoming Headaches and Migraines:

"A complete and understandable guide for both the practitioner and the patient...Lisa Morrone's extensive preparation, research, and years of experience are reflected in the safe and clinically proven techniques she recommends. A must-read for primary and specialty providers... and of course, anyone who suffers from headaches."

—William Robert Spencer, MD, FAAP
ear, nose, and throat specialist

Overcoming Back and Neck Pain:

"Unique—it enables the nonmedical person to understand and manage their pain, but it is comprehensive enough to be an excellent resource and reference guide for physicians who take care of these problems. Well done."

—Warwick Green. MD,
orthopedic surgeon

"A very practical approach to the key things patients really need to know. I recommend it to all sufferers from spine problems...I appreciate Lisa's treatment of every person as someone who has not only a body and mind, but a spirit as well."

—Kent Keyser, MS, PT, OCS, COMT, ATC, FFCFMT, FAAOMPT,
practicing and teaching physical therapist

"A treasure chest of information, easily understood, and presented with clarity, wit, and optimism...a truly enjoyable journey from head to toe. A definite re-read!"

—Mary G. Flanagan, RPA, physician assistant
Adjunct Professor, Touro College PA Program

Overcoming Overeating

Lisa Morrone, PT

HARVEST HOUSE PUBLISHERS

EUGENE, OREGON

Cover by Dugan Design Group, Bloomington, Minnesota

Cover photos © DNY 59 / iStockphoto; Oleg Prikhodko / iStockphoto; Amy Walters / Fotolia

Graphics of addiction cycle by Peter Morrone; back-cover author photo © Peter Morrone

Published in association with the William K. Jensen Literary Agency, 119 Bampton Court, Eugene, Oregon 97404.

This book is not intended to take the place of sound professional medical advice. Neither the author nor the publisher assumes any liability for possible adverse consequences as a result of the information contained herein.

OVERCOMING OVEREATING
Copyright © 2009 by Lisa Morrone, P.T.
Published by Harvest House Publishers
Eugene, Oregon 97402
www.harvesthousepublishers.com

Library of Congress Cataloging-in-Publication Data
    Morrone, Lisa, 1967-
    Overcoming overeating / Lisa Morrone.
       p. cm.
    Includes bibliographical references.
    ISBN 978-0-7369-2702-4 (pbk.)
    1. Compulsive eating—Popular works. I. Title.
    RC552.C65M675 2009
    616.85'26—dc22

                              2009017209

Printed in the United States of America

09 10 11 12 13 14 15 16 17 / VP-SK / 10 9 8 7 6 5 4 3 2 1

It is not good to eat too much...
A person without self-control is like
a city whose walls are broken down.

—PROVERBS 25:28

Acknowledgments

Without a doubt, the first person I must thank is my literary agent, Bill Jensen, who upon reading the subtitle I had written for another book, *It's Not What You Eat, It's What Eats You*, thought it would make a wonderful book title as well as a desperately needed, fresh look at the subject of weight loss. I followed his advice, as did the publisher's committee at Harvest House, and voilà, this book was born.

My heart is full of admiration and gratitude for my editor, Paul Gossard, at Harvest House Publishers. Paul, this is our third book together (with more on the way). Your encouragement, attention to detail, and your eloquent mastery of the English language, along with your constant attention to the reader, have polished my writing, once again, to a high gloss! I am so thankful Harvest House paired us together.

I am always mindful of the risk that the publisher's committee took on this new author back in 2006. To Terry Glaspey, LaRae Weikert, Bob Hawkins Jr., John Constance, and Barb Sherrill: I am honored to partner with you each in book publishing. I have found a comfortable home with a warm family. Thank you for your continued enthusiasm in my book writing.

Special thanks to Scott Forsmith, CSW, who has read this manuscript in its entirety and has added to its effectiveness with his wisdom of patient care in the field of psychology.

I would be remiss not to thank those of you who have shared your personal journeys within the pages of this book. Your candid reflections are a true encouragement. May your stories resonate with the hearts of many who struggle, as you did, with food addiction.

Also, much love and gratitude goes out to my RYT Prayer Team. Ladies, you faithfully undergird all I do. With your support, God is able to do "immeasurably more than all we ask or imagine."

Lastly, I must give credit for this book's completeness to my husband, Peter Morrone, who for the third time now has read and critiqued each chapter I have written three times over! Your input has blessed me and my readers alike (and probably made my editor's job a bit easier!). *I love you, always.*

CONTENTS

Foreword

by Ron Eaker, MD

The world needs another diet book about as much as it needs another flu pandemic, so it's a good thing Lisa Morrone didn't write one! *Overcoming Overeating* is a lifeline thrown to the millions of people who struggle with their weight. As a practicing physician for over 20 years, I have seen firsthand the devastation of being "overfat." Men and women dramatically reduce both the quantity and quality of their years as they are forced to deal with the side effects of overweight and obesity: hypertension, diabetes, stroke, cancer, depression, and more.

Overcoming Overeating acknowledges the medical and mental destruction that comes from weight that's out of control, but it provides hope that springs from Lisa's grasp of the nature of obesity—a disorder involving mind, body, and spirit. With her personal and professional experience saturating the pages, she succinctly outlines a plan to help you jump off the "not-so-merry-go-round," as she calls it.

Weight control is 75 percent above the neck. It is a brain game, and to win the game you have to understand both how and why you play. Dr. John Sklare, a friend and a noted weight-loss author, states, "To change your weight, you have to change your mind!" Lisa attacks this problem at its core, laying out a practical, sustainable, and results-oriented approach that will guide you to permanent mind change. Most important, she incorporates the wisdom and guidance of Scripture, pointing you to grace and forgiveness...two concepts you won't find in many weight-loss books.

One of the key principles of Lisa's program is that knowledge by itself is not power—rather, it's the *application* of knowledge that yields sustained success. As part of this process she introduces you to the stories and successes of many real-life people. Their journeys will inspire and motivate you because they too have struggled with their weight.

As a physician, author, and dad, would I recommend this book to patients and family members? I would not only recommend it—for some of you I feel it may be your best hope for dealing with the mental and emotional side of overeating. Viktor Frankl said, "If you know the why, the how will follow." *Overcoming Overeating* provides both the why and the how toward becoming the new, healthy you.

—J. Ron Eaker, MD
Physician and author of *Fat-Proof Your Family* and
A Woman's Guide to Hormone Health

Overcoming Overeating

Waist Management

Food is not the problem.

May I ask you a personal question right off the bat? How many attempts at dieting have you made over your lifetime?

If you're holding this book, I'm pretty sure your answer lies somewhere between 5 and 25. That is, if you can even recall every time you said to yourself, *Enough is enough! I've got to do something about my weight*—and then set out methodically to "go on a diet." Maybe some of your dieting attempts were successful—for a time. But then, over the next year or two, you slowly regained what you lost in the first place. Worse yet, maybe you gained back every pound and then some!

The worst part of dieting, even worse than the restrictions of the diet itself, is the eventual failure…and the intense guilt you feel when you've "broken your diet"…and the consuming (pardon the pun) feeling of not having the necessary willpower to ever succeed. (*Who is this Will Power anyway? And why is it that he must be present in order for a diet to work for you?* We'll talk more about him later.) Yet every time a new diet comes on the market, you buy the book or join the club and try, try again…only to be met once more by frustration, guilt, and perhaps even self-ridicule and condemnation for having failed yet again.

What went wrong for you the last time around? You made sure you were well-educated on the plan you'd chosen. You filled your home with all the allowable foodstuffs. Maybe you joined a support group. You had specific goals and good intentions, and once again you invited Mr. Will Power to join you. Even with all this in place, failure eventually came. After living through this cycle of diet-failure-diet-failure for the umpteenth time, you've come to the conclusion it isn't the diets' fault—it's *your* fault. You are unsuccessful at dieting.

Now before you get too down on yourself, I believe that, unknowingly, you began each of your past diets at a severe disadvantage. You were never properly prepared for successful "waist management."

❦

Allow me to explain. I believe the primary reason you haven't had success with dieting is because *most overeating is a symptom of what lies deep within your heart, mind, and soul.* Your heart is the seat of your *emotions*, both positive and negative feelings. Like it or not, your emotions have a strong effect on all you do (or don't do). Your mind is where your *thoughts* live, both the ones you are conscious of and those that sneak around undetected in your subconscious. What you think about yourself and the world around you is very powerful. Finally, your soul is that eternal vessel that longs to be filled with *spiritual* food. Upon investigation, you may find yourself to be spiritually empty.

While I agree with a number of the weight-loss plans and programs available today, I strongly believe that weight loss is not simply about food balancing and portion control. It must begin with an initial assessment of the *person* who is attempting to lose weight—not merely the food they will eat or not eat. This assessment needs to include not only a physical baseline, but also an emotional, mental, and spiritual evaluation as well. Repair and strengthening of each of these aspects will lay the critical foundation upon which weight loss and, ultimately, healthy weight maintenance can be built. Not preparing (and repairing) yourself in these areas *before* beginning a dietary life change is like attempting to install new windows in your house without fixing the rot in the existing wooden frames. There's likely nothing wrong with the new windows (the diet) you've chosen, but your home (your entire self) is not "healthy" enough to accept the upgrade.

And what about that guy Will Power anyway? Well, *his* strength and effectiveness depend upon *your* healthy thoughts and emotions. You can invite him to help you while you work on your new consumption plan…but as time passes, if you continue to feed him a diet of unhealthy thoughts and painful emotions, Mr. Power will become increasingly weak. When ultimately his health begins to fail, you "slip"…"break your diet"…"fall off the food wagon"—by making a high-calorie decision, and you seal his fate. No more Mr. Will Power.

Die-t or Live-it Plan?

Can we replace the term *diet* with something better? I've always hated the word. I think it's because it contains the word *die*, which has such negative connotations! I much prefer a term I came across years ago…so let's agree from this time forward to call a well-balanced food and lifestyle modification effort a *live-it* plan. Absurd plans that require eating grapefruits at each meal or such we can still refer to as die-ts—because that's no way to live!

I'm sure you're frustrated with your lack of dieting success. I am right there with you. It frustrates and saddens me to watch my patients, friends, and family members yo-yo their body weight up and down and starve themselves in order to move the arrow on their bathroom scales to the left. And all the while their daily food intake causes their self-esteem to rise and go down like the sun. Don't get me wrong— I'm a proponent of weight-loss methods and of making food and lifestyle changes that will improve your overall health. But if you try to follow a diet plan without first healing your mind (your thought life), your heart (your emotions), and your soul (your spirit), you are doomed to fail, simply because your foundation needs to be repaired beforehand.

≈❦≈

If what I'm saying is resonating with you, then you will certainly find new hope and promise in this book. As its cover states: "Finally, a weight loss book *without* a diet plan!" Here you'll find the tools you need to evaluate your heart, mind, and soul. These are followed by well-tested, tried-and-true methods to break the cycle of food addiction from the *inside out*—because *food* is not the problem!

When you begin to understand and address the underlying causes of your overeating, you'll no longer find yourself using food as a time-filler, mood-elevator, or painkiller. You'll be freed to achieve steady, lasting results using any reputable diet. You'll be able to live a life that enables you to make healthy food decisions.

Chapter 1

Putting on the Pounds

Take stock of your situation.

In the introduction to this book we spoke of the critical importance of making a personal assessment pre-diet (or rather, pre-*live*-it plan). To be effective, the assessment must consider the areas we've already mentioned: 1) physical, 2) emotional, 3) mental, and 4) spiritual. The first and most obvious of these four components is physical appraisal, this chapter's subject.

It has been my experience as a health-care practitioner that many of my patients have an inaccurate view of how much extra weight they are actually carrying. For instance, some of you may have always thought you needed to lose weight, even when those around you didn't agree. You struggle on diets, always trying to achieve your desired "target weight"—yet your target is based on personal preference, not on science. You've never actually investigated what your healthy weight range should be. All you know is you want to be a size 6.

This discrepancy can stem from not being satisfied with your God-given body type. (You hate the hips your mother gave you, or you despise your father's pot belly, which began to show up around your waistline a few years ago.) You constantly compare your body with the bodies of the models and actors you see each day in print, on the TV, online, and in the movies. (Many of these, by the way, are clinically underweight or struggling with anorexia.) Although you may be absolutely correct that you have *some* weight to shed, your expectations of where you should be don't necessarily line up with the weight charts provided by the medical world.

Others of you have a more casual view of your size. *Yeah, I need to lose a good 20 pounds*, you admit to yourself. In actuality, if you were to weigh and measure yourself and consult a weight chart, you need to lose more like 40 pounds! Neither of these people has an accurate idea of where their present body weight places them on a chart, nor are they aware of what their target weight range should be. An honest physical self-assessment is the first step in your recovery process. Without it, everything is left to a good guess, or a poor guesstimate!

Overweight or Obese?

Before we go about actually weighing, measuring, and sizing you up, let's talk first about what information we are looking to obtain. There are specific terms used in medical literature to describe the amount a person weighs. The first is *underweight*—a state in which the body is maintained at a lower-than-healthy weight. Risks here arise from such things as hormonal imbalances caused by low body-fat content and increased risk of hip fractures among the aged. Elderly people often fall into this category because their muscle mass, and therefore body weight, begins to decline as they age. Anorexics also fall into this category. If extreme, they lose their life to this illness.

The second term, which should be your ultimate goal, is to be of *normal* body weight. Normal weight is actually a *range* that allows for differing body types (small, medium, or large frames), sex (male or female), and ranges of body-fat content (22 to 25 percent for women; 15 to 18 percent for men).

You also may find that your results will place you into one of two further categories: *overweight* or *obese*. *Overweight* is the "diagnosis" when a person's body weight is anywhere from 1 to 19 percent greater than their suggested weight range. For example, a person of either sex whose height is five-foot-nine would be considered overweight if he or she weighed 1 to 34 pounds beyond their normal range of 125 to

169. So if you're five-foot-nine, weighing anywhere between 170 to 204 pounds would qualify you as being overweight.

Muscle Mass

When muscular athletes compare their body weight and height measurement ratios with what is considered *normal,* they usually fall within the range of *overweight.* This is simply due to the fact that their muscles, which weigh more than fat, place them inaccurately high on the weight charts. Remember, these weight suggestions are based on a *typical* distribution of fat vs. muscle. And athletes are anything but typical when it comes to their muscles.

The next term, used to describe the *extremely* overweight population, is *obese.* We are hearing a lot more about obesity in the media nowadays. That is because the number of people in our nation in this category continues to rise at an alarming rate. Formerly, only a handful of states were facing a high percentage of population obesity—now, our nation is experiencing an obesity epidemic! (See the progression in the maps below.)

Percent of Obesity in U.S. Adults

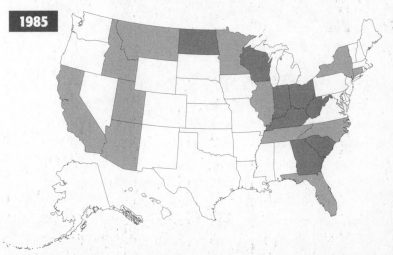

1985

□ No Data   ▨ <10%   ▨ 10%-14%   ▨ 15%-19%   ▨ 20%-24%   ■ 25%-29%   ■ >30%

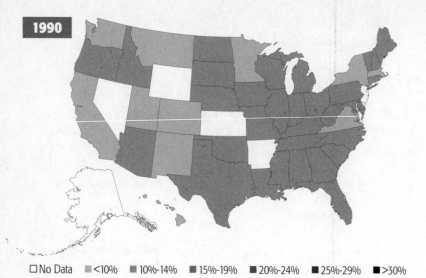

□ No Data   ■ <10%   ■ 10%-14%   ■ 15%-19%   ■ 20%-24%   ■ 25%-29%   ■ >30%

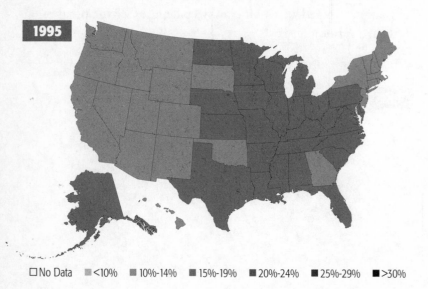

□ No Data   ■ <10%   ■ 10%-14%   ■ 15%-19%   ■ 20%-24%   ■ 25%-29%   ■ >30%

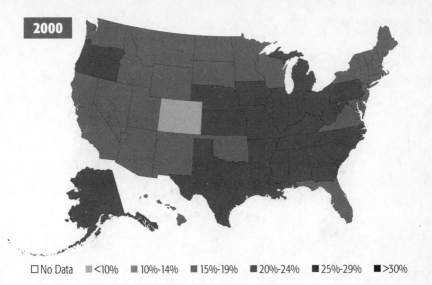

2000

☐ No Data ■ <10% ■ 10%-14% ■ 15%-19% ■ 20%-24% ■ 25%-29% ■ >30%

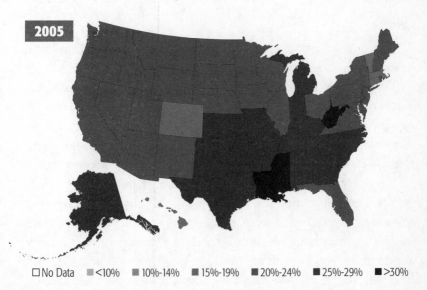

2005

☐ No Data ■ <10% ■ 10%-14% ■ 15%-19% ■ 20%-24% ■ 25%-29% ■ >30%

And in just two more years...

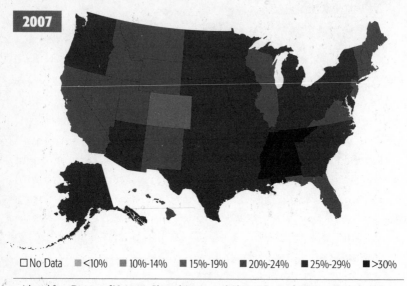

2007

☐ No Data   ▨ <10%   ■ 10%-14%   ■ 15%-19%   ■ 20%-24%   ■ 25%-29%   ■ >30%

Adapted from Division of Nutrition, Physical Activity and Obesity, Centers for Disease Control and Prevention, "U.S. Obesity Rates 1985-2007," July 24, 2008, www.cdc.gov/nccdphp/dnpa/obesity/trend/maps/index.htm.

Aren't those statistics shocking? Obesity is nothing short of a wildfire sweeping across our nation. And people's lives are being burned up!

Do you know if *you* fit into this weight category? If you've answered, "Yes," I'm sure you remember the day your doctor first "labeled you." It was quite an emotional blow, wasn't it? Even though those maps clearly show that you are among a vast number of others in our country, let's face it—no one suffers obesity issues "in groups." It is a lonely fight.

On the other hand, you may have no idea where your overweight puts you on the continuum. By the end of this chapter you may discover, for the very first time, that the term *obesity* does in fact describe you. When your body weight is 20 percent greater than your healthy weight range, you have moved from *overweight* into the *obese* category. And with it, your health risks have markedly increased (see chapter 2 for specifics). In order for you to have a specific example of what obesity "looks" like, consider again someone whose height is five-foot-nine. They would be considered obese if they weighed in excess of 205 pounds (greater than 36 pounds over the high point of their acceptable weight range).

In recent years, physicians have been taking the obesity diagnosis to a new level, that of *morbidly obese*. Morbid obesity, by definition, describes a person who weighs 50 to 100 percent, or more than 100 pounds, over their ideal weight range. Many physicians are now becoming quite forthright with their patients, telling them they are *morbidly* obese (rather than just obese). If you have received this upsetting report, don't get angry at your doctor. He or she is simply trying to jump-start a crisis intervention in your own heart and mind. Health risks from this degree of obesity are so severe that they are morbid, or deadly. According to the National Institute of Health's Consensus Report, morbid obesity has become a serious chronic disease in the United States. Today, of the 97 million Americans who are overweight or obese, an estimated 5 to 10 million are considered morbidly obese. In fact:

> *More than one-third of the adult population in*
> *the United States is presently overweight or obese.*

So What's in a Pound?

When you look back through your childhood pictures, can you pinpoint a time when you noticed your "fat" occurring? Or were you a chubby little kid from the get-go? What about your teenage or college years? Did you put on the "freshman 10" (pounds, that is), or possibly the "freshman 20 or 30"? Maybe the extra weight you're carrying piled on when you were "all grown up"—when you began your first stressful job, or after the birth of your first child or, sadly, at the end of your marriage. Perhaps you cannot pinpoint an exact time. But each year you weigh more than the year before. Regardless of why or when "fat" happened, pounds have been added to your frame, and now the life you've always pictured no longer fits into that frame.

Each extra, unwanted pound, though it may sit on a different location on your body, is structurally the same. Those pounds are made up of *adipose* tissue (fat cells), which became "stuffed" because of excess calorie consumption. Even though you are growing fatter, you are not growing more fat cells. The cells you have are simply getting stuffed—just like eating more doesn't increase the number of stomachs you have, it simply stuffs the one you do have! In order to gain one pound, you had to have eaten 3500 calories beyond what your body needed. And because "fair's fair" in the battle of the bulge, in order to rid your body of that pound, you must use, or "burn off," approximately 3500 more calories than you take in.

Calories Defined

Diet-savvy people talk all the time about how many calories a food has in it, how many calories one should eat or not eat each day, and how many calories are burned up doing a particular activity. But does anyone actually know what a calorie is?

A calorie (cal) is a measure of energy in the form of *heat* (not a measure of fat, as some believe it to be). One *food* calorie (1 kcal, which is actually equal to 1000 regular calories) is the amount of food energy (heat) needed to raise the temperature of 1 kilogram of water 1 degree Celsius. Food sources are turned into this caloric food energy via the digestion process.

The way in which calorie counts are determined (and then posted on your food packaging or in calorie charts) is quite interesting. The food in question is set ablaze. The amount of heat energy required to completely obliterate it is measured. The heat energy (or calories) used is noted—and voilà, you know how many food calories are in that bacon double cheeseburger!

Not all foods are created equal. Foods we eat or drink can be classified as either protein, carbohydrates, fat, or a combination of these. One gram of a protein or carbohydrate will release four calories of energy when digested, whereas one gram of fat will produce nine calories. Therefore, gram per gram, fats are a richer potential energy (calorie) source than proteins or carbohydrates. That said, it is incorrect to believe that *only* fatty foods make you fat.

Now here's the real reason why the pounds begin to rack up: After you eat or drink a food item, all of its "digestive energy" will be released into your bloodstream in the form of glucose (sugar molecules)—regardless of whether it started off as a protein, carbohydrate, or fat. If your intake has supplied more circulating energy (glucose) than is needed at the present time, your body will store this energy away for a future need, should one arise (which in our abundantly fed and underexercised culture rarely does).

The storage tanks your body uses for all that excess energy are called fat cells. Digested foods that have been reduced into glucose molecules within your bloodstream are next converted into glycogen molecules. These excess glycogen molecules are then picked up from your bloodstream and are put away for "safekeeping" in your fat cells. If overeating continues, more and more energy (excess glucose/glycogen) is stored away, and your fat cells become increasingly stuffed and "puffy," adding to the roundness of your body.

How Do You Measure Up?

There are three excellent methods to determine which weight category you're in. From them you can determine your associated disease-based risk factors.

1. Body Mass Index

The first method is called the *body mass index*, or BMI. A mathematical calculation is made using your height and your weight to determine your category.

You can calculate this number for yourself. All you'll need is a pencil and clean notebook—we will be using this notebook throughout the course of this book, so make sure it has plenty of pages left! (For those of you who ran screaming from your math classroom when a student, simply go to my Web site, www.RestoringYourTemple.com, and click on the "BMI Calculator" button.) Okay, now go step on your scale. I mean it—no good will come from a mere guess. It's time to get real with yourself and your weight issue.

Okay, here goes: Plug in your height (in inches) and your weight (in pounds), and your BMI number will be calculated.

$$BMI = \frac{(\text{ Weight in pounds }) \times 703}{(\text{Height in inches}) \times (\text{Height in inches})}$$

For example, a person who weighs 170 pounds and is five-foot-three will have a BMI of 30.1:

$$\frac{(170 \text{ pounds}) \times 703}{(63 \text{ inches}) \times (63 \text{ inches})}$$

BMI = 30.1

Now look to the chart below to determine your true weight status. As I said before, this method does not have separate charts for men and women.

BMI	Weight status
Below 18.5	Underweight
18.5–24.9	Normal
25.0–29.9	Overweight
30.0 and above	Obese

I'm sorry if your discovery brings pain…but there is no hope for your recovery without beginning at the point of truth. I hope you will keep your eyes focused, as mine are, toward the future. I'm looking forward to a new day for you—a day when you will no longer feel embarrassed when you step on a scale or into a dressing room. Good things are in store for you if you dedicate yourself to the recovery plan set forth in this book.

2. Waist Circumference

The second method for determining your weight-related health risks requires a measurement of the circumference of your waist. According to the National Heart, Lung, and Blood Institute, waist circumference is a good indicator of abdominal fat, which is another predictor of your risk for developing some potentially deadly diseases. (We'll thoroughly discuss those risks in the next chapter.)

Here's how to take the next measurement. Use a flexible tape measure and wrap it around your midsection (no shirt required), just above your hip bones. For accuracy, begin and end at your belly button. If your tape measure doesn't make it all the way around your middle, simply mark your skin with a pen and measure again from there, adding the full length of the original tape measure to the extra inches you needed to complete a full "lap" around. Now refer to the chart below to determine your risk status based upon both your BMI and the circumference of your waist.

Risk of Associated Disease According to BMI and Waist Size			
BMI	Weight category	Waist less than or equal to 40 inches (men) or 35 inches (women)	Waist greater than 40 inches (men) or 35 inches (women)
18.5 or less	Underweight	–	N/A
18.5–24.9	Normal	–	N/A
25.0–29.9	**Overweight**	**Increased**	**High**
30.0–34.9	Obese	High	Very high
35.0–39.9	**Obese**	**Very high**	**Very high**
40 or greater	Extremely obese	Extremely high	Extremely high

If your BMI is greater than 25, the National Heart, Lung, and Blood Institute recommends losing weight—particularly if you have a high waist measurement (greater than 40 inches for men and 35 inches for women) or if you know you have other risk factors for disease (see the next chapter). Even a loss of only 10 percent of your current weight will lower your risk of developing diseases associated with obesity. If you are overweight (BMI>25) but *don't* have a high waist measurement and have fewer than two other risk factors, you may simply need to prevent further weight gain rather than actually lose weight. Now there's some good news!

3. Waist-to-Hip Ratio

The third simple scientific method used to determine your health-risk status vis-à-vis your weight is called the *waist-to-hip ratio,* or WHR. Once

again you'll need a tape measure, pen and paper, and possibly a calculator. If you've been actively following along to this point, you already
have your waist measurement to plug into the equation below. In order to
get the last bit of data, simply take the same "round the body" measurement, but this time run the tape measure around the *widest part* of your
hips. Now I understand that this final measurement is not a comfortable one for many of you women—honestly, who can get excited about
measuring their buttocks and hips? Many of you will be glad to know
that the larger your hip-buttocks circumference is relative to your waist,
the *less* your projected health risk is. So big smiles here for those who are
"pear-shaped."

To calculate your WHR, simply *divide your waist measurement by
your hip measurement.*

For example:

Waist circumference = 40 inches

Hip circumference = 38 inches

Waist-to-hip-ratio = 40 ÷ 38 = *1.05,*
which according to the chart below is high risk.

The number you end up with correlates with your associated health
risk status (see chart below), according to Dr. Devendra Singh, a psychologist who developed this method back in 1993 while at the University of
Texas. As a result of her research, it was determined that optimal WHR
for women is *.7,* and for men, *.9.*

Waist-to-Hip Ratio Chart		
Male	Female	Health risk based solely on WHR
0.95 or below	0.80 or below	Low risk
0.96 to 1.0	0.81 to 0.85	Moderate risk
1.0+	0.85+	High risk

Interestingly, WHR has been found to be a more efficient predictor of mortality in older people than waist circumference or body mass index.[1] And if obesity were to be redefined using WHR instead of BMI, the proportion of people categorized as at risk of heart attack worldwide would increase threefold![2]

Your Starting Point

So which method should you use to determine your weight category and risk factor? I believe you should consider the results from all three (BMI, BMI with waist measurement, and WHR). This way you will get a comprehensive picture of where you are today. In other words, you will be able to place a well-defined "You Are Here" arrow to mark your starting point on this path away from remaining overweight. As you journey toward taking back the control food has had over your life, you *must* be willing to take an honest look at all the factors involved before you can make any lasting improvements. A reality check is never easy, but there will never be recovery without it.

Chapter 2

The High Cost of Overweight

*Some things aren't worth
the price you've had to pay.*

Sometimes we lose perspective on how much something costs us simply because we pay that cost little by little, over a long period of time. Take a home mortgage, for instance. When you take out a $150,000 loan to purchase your first home, it seems more palatable (and less frightening) after the bank breaks the ginormous sum down into 360 "easy payments" for you, to be made monthly over a 30-year period. All you see is your monthly bill of maybe $1200, rather than the big picture. Truth is—when all is said and done, and repaid—you actually owe your lender well over $300,000!

Likewise, when it comes to the costs you endure for being overweight or obese, you've likely protected yourself by refusing to look at the whole picture—it's just too overwhelming. So each day or month you allow yourself to acknowledge only a small portion of the total cost, such as, *I just can't find a dress for this wedding, because there's so little selection in my size*, or, *They gave my promotion away to that skinny guy!*

There are numerous social and employment costs as well as health risks associated with being overweight or obese. These costs are quite serious. Whenever I find I must confront a friend about a serious matter, my tone changes from light and easy to more serious and focused. Please understand this if you notice my tone has changed somewhat. I'm delivering this message with love and care. Yet it's so very important that I don't want to candy-coat it in any way or present it in a lighthearted manner. Obviously, your personal risks and costs increase the larger your body becomes. Once you clearly understand all the costs involved, you can decide for yourself whether you are willing to continue paying them.

It's time to stop protecting yourself. This chapter provides you with the complete "cost analysis" of being overweight in order to bring you to the point of being concerned and regretful enough to make a choice—to decide you cannot and will not spend another day of your life held captive by fat and food. Some of the costs you'll encounter here may be ones you've been refusing to face for years.

To improve the effectiveness of this chapter, I suggest you pick up the notebook you began using in the last chapter. Write down each cost you are presently paying or have paid in the past—all the while taking stock of all that your food issues will likely cost you in the future. Are you ready to get real with yourself?

Who Is *That* Person in the Mirror?

You and I live not only in a society that places high value on physical beauty, but also in a time in history where the definition of beauty seems to have become awfully *thin*, wouldn't you agree? When you look at paintings from the Renaissance, women, partially clothed, had—to put it plainly—"rolls." Rounded figures were the rage. Not so today. We are continually assaulted with skeletally gaunt girls slinking up and down fashion runways, and men whose unclothed chests boast of many hours in the gym lifting weights. Wow, who can compete with that?

Though you and I may never measure up to the distorted beauty standards of the day, we all have a desire to be considered attractive to some degree by another person (not including our mothers). When you became overweight or obese, you may have cost yourself the joy and satisfaction of making someone's head turn or heart skip a beat.

Maybe *you* are turned off by your own reflection in the mirror. When a person feels physically attractive, they gain a sense of self-confidence—and this may be something you haven't felt in quite some time. So if the problem of lost attractiveness hits home, chalk it up as one of the costs you've had to endure from being overweight.

It's a Small World After All...

Many of you would agree that your world is much smaller than you'd like it to be. Sure, your family accepts you, and for the most part you feel safe around them. But a party or an after-hours office get-together...well, then your hands begin to sweat, and you try to come up with a believable excuse why you must decline the invitation. *Why would they want me there anyway?* you think to yourself. Even if you do force yourself to venture out, you are uneasy around all that food and all those eyes. You just know people are watching you, waiting to see how much food you'll eat. So you eat next to nothing just to prove them wrong. Then you go home and eat everything in sight, in private.

Be honest with yourself. Do you, or have you in the past, shut out potential friends, love interests, or even the enjoyment of social events because of your weight issues? *Why would anyone want to be friends with a fat boy?* you've asked yourself as a teenager, quickly agreeing with yourself that *of course, no one would!*

But that's only half the story. How many people have passed *you* by, falsely believing you wouldn't be a good friend or life partner, simply based on your mass and nothing else? People can be cruel. And fat jokes and taunting have been the lot of many of you from the early days of the playground to grown-up days at the office. The social cost of overweight can be devastating. If you've experienced it, write it down as well.

Hi-Ho, Hi-Ho, It's Off to Work I Go

Job interviews are difficult for you, aren't they? Maybe that's why you've stayed in the same job beyond the time you should have left. You know you can do more, can look for a better position elsewhere, but the thought of sitting before an interviewer in "this state" is so upsetting that you simply stay put.

The reason you feel this way is not irrational. It's quite rational. Numerous studies have shown that in the employment world, people hold prejudices against those who are significantly overweight.[1] Such studies have long revealed that society judges overweight or obese people to be

- lazy
- undisciplined
- not conscientious
- less intelligent
- lacking good hygiene
- sloppy and disorganized
- emotionally unstable
- unbalanced

Even those who are overweight themselves report the same prejudices about their peers who are overweight or obese.

It's my experience with friends, family members, and patients alike that none of these prejudices hold true. No more so than in the normal-to-underweight population. But studies confirm that, on average, overweight persons are hired less, promoted less often, and salaried lower than their thinner counterparts.[2] If you've experienced one or more of these workplace costs...write them down. You need to prove to yourself that this overeating thing costs too much to continue!

The *Inner* Truth About Overweight

Whether or not you want to look at it this way, the reality is that you are slowly committing suicide by remaining overweight. The excessive food you put into your mouth is having a poisoning effect on the organs and systems of your body. *Being obese decreases your life expectancy by 7 years.* If you also smoke, you are cutting your life short by *13 to 15 years.*[3]

This cost definitely has my attention because it falls so close to home for me. Both of my parents struggled with being overweight (and at times, clinically obese) most of their adult lives. Each experienced childhood and adulthood issues that were never resolved, only suppressed. Neither one pursued healing or release from their angst. My father lived his life in a near continuous state of overweight, with the exception of an occasional six-to-eight-month diet/weight loss/resume unhealthy eating/regain the lost weight sort of thing. You know what I'm talking about. At the age of 55, he had his first major heart attack, losing the function of most of the front wall of his heart. Four years later, his emotional pain still unaddressed and his lifestyle unchanged, he experienced his last, sudden, fatal heart attack.

My mother, who readily admitted that she held onto pain from her past, used food both as a tranquilizer and an anger-management "tool" (or should I say, "stuffer"). As a result, at least partly, she suffered with her own health issues, such as high blood pressure and early dementia—both of which have ties to being overweight. These conditions began to develop in her early sixties, decades before they should have. I want desperately to help you spare yourself, your children, and your loved ones this awful pain of loss that results from your misuse of food.

So that you'll know exactly what you are risking, the following is a laundry list of health ailments known to be caused by overweight and obesity. Again, if you are going to set your feet solidly on the starting line of recovery, you need to know all that you are running away from, as well as what you are running toward. As Beth Moore says in her book *Stepping Up*, "Sometimes the best motivation we'll ever have for going someplace new is distress over someplace old."

Metabolic Syndrome

Here's an obesity-related health problem you're probably not familiar with. Actually it is a *group* of five risk factors (many of which you will recognize) that correlate highly with the presence of *cardiovascular disease* and with *type 2 diabetes* (see sidebar).[4] Included are

- *Altered levels and ratios of fat substances (lipids) in your bloodstream*, specifically high levels of cholesterol and triglycerides, decreased high-density lipoproteins (HDLs—the "good cholesterol"), and elevated low-density lipoproteins (LDLs—the "bad cholesterol").

- *High blood pressure.*
- *High blood-sugar levels* (often with associated insulin resistance—we'll get to that in a moment).
- *Increased risk of clotting* (a pro-thrombotic state).
- *Heightened inflammation* (a.k.a. a pro-inflammatory state).

Cardiovascular disease encompasses numerous diseases that affect the heart or blood vessels. Some examples are heart attack (myocardial infarction), stroke (cerebral vascular accident), high blood pressure (hypertension), and "hardening of the arteries" (atherosclerosis).

Type 2 diabetes is a condition characterized by high blood-sugar levels caused by either a lack of insulin production within the pancreas or the body's inability to use insulin efficiently (*insulin resistance*). Often the result of obesity, type 2 diabetes, which used to be an adult-onset disease, is now affecting an increasing number of children as well. Complications are numerous. They include increased cardiovascular risks, blindness, nerve damage, and kidney disease.

Let me explain in broad strokes the processes and subsequent dangers these five conditions pose. The better you understand what's happening to your body when you're overweight, the more motivated you'll be to leave that state behind.

1. Altered and elevated levels of circulating fats (lipids) abrade the smooth walls of your blood vessels, much like pebbles flowing through your water pipes would begin to wear down their insides. Your body's response to these abrasions is inflammation (swelling), and repair of the damage by importing other cells (macrophages) and ultimately by laying down more smooth muscle cells. Both of these processes cause your blood vessels to narrow. Lipids (LDLs and triglycerides) can also adhere to these inflamed areas, further narrowing and subsequently obstructing blood flow. HDLs (the "good" cholesterol) help carry LDLs away from the walls of blood vessels and return them to the bloodstream, thus preventing buildup of cholesterol in the walls. When HDL levels drop below 40mg/dl, you lose that anticlogging benefit.

2. High blood pressure (hypertension) (HTN) increases the turbulence (or speed and agitation) of the blood flowing through your vessels. A higher rate of blood flow creates more internal damage from abrasive circulating substances (lipids and even blood cells themselves). Blood pressure is considered to be clinically high when greater than 130/85 mmHg. Hypertension increases your risk of suffering, or dying as a result of, a stroke—the brain's version of a heart attack. Over time, hypertension can also lead to congestive heart failure and kidney damage or failure.

3. High blood-sugar levels are a big problem. The higher your blood-sugar levels get, the thicker your blood becomes. Thicker blood moves through your vessels more slowly and takes a much greater effort by your heart to pump it, putting you at increased risk for heart attack and stroke. A normal blood sugar should be 100mg/dl (or "100" for simplicity's sake). If your levels go beyond 500, your blood takes on the consistency of the heavy syrup in a can of peaches! Try pumping *that* through your tiny capillaries!

What causes your sugar levels to become high in the first place? They're normally controlled and maintained by the production of *insulin*, which is released from your pancreas into your bloodstream. *Insulin receptors* in your muscles, liver, and fat cells respond by accepting circulating sugar molecules for storage. (Insulin is the key that unlocks the receptors, sort of like a lock-and-key mechanism.) This mechanism is ultimately responsible for regulating your metabolism. In a healthy human, insulin levels (which respond to the amount of sugar present in your bloodstream) establish how much sugar will be left in circulation and how much will be stored in your body's organs. It is no understatement to say that you and I owe our lives to this sensitive mechanism! Too little blood sugar and you'll die; too much—again, you'll die.

This feedback mechanism becomes unbalanced in persons who are overweight (especially those who have a higher percentage of abdominal fat). Overeating provides a steady overabundance of available blood sugar. To meet the high demand, insulin production efforts are increased. Because the insulin receptors are constantly being inundated with high amounts of insulin, they tend to lose their sensitivity to insulin. (Sort of like a mother who hears her child call, "Mommy, mommy" for the hundredth time tends to tune them out.) The receptors, which should respond to the presence of circulating insulin by pulling excess sugar out of your bloodstream, instead remain in a "locked" state. The result is consistently higher circulating blood-sugar levels.

This condition is known as *insulin resistance,* which is now understood to be *the* cause of every component of metabolic syndrome. If not addressed with dietary changes, insulin resistance will eventually become type 2 diabetes (you've moved from insulin-resistant to "insulin-defiant").* Type 2 diabetes is not your friend! As mentioned in the sidebar, it increases your risk of heart attack (upwards of tenfold) and can lead to blindness and neuropathy (loss of sensation, nerve-generated pain, or both), among other dreadful things.

The Sugar–Fat Connection

Insulin resistance, caused primarily by overeating foods laden with refined carbohydrates and sugars, also affects the liver's ability to absorb and store fats from your bloodstream, thus increasing your triglyceride and LDL levels. More bad news for your cardiovascular system!

4. Increased risk of clotting (a pro-thrombotic state) is harmful for the simple reason that a clot inside an artery is a bad thing. If it occurs in a limb, you can lose the limb. If it occurs in your heart, you'll experience an "oxygen and food" shortage in your heart, and a heart attack can result. And if it occurs within your brain, you've just "stroked out"!

Many years ago I treated a patient who was an overweight smoker. Although she was in physical therapy for a neck issue, she complained that her left hand always felt cold. Whenever I felt her hand, I never detected a temperature difference between it and her right hand—until one particular day. It was so very cold that I immediately took her pulse at her wrist—that is, I *attempted* to take her pulse. It was not there!

---

* Interestingly, exercise has been found to reverse this loss of insulin sensitivity in muscle tissue.[5]

I immediately sent her to her doctor, who had to perform emergency surgery to unblock an artery. She returned to physical therapy the next week with a surgical bandage across the lower left side of her neck and a smile across her face. The timely diagnosis and emergency surgery had saved her arm! Close call...too close for both of us. It is never good to continue with an eating lifestyle that increases your susceptibility to clotting.

5. Heightened inflammation (a pro-inflammatory state) is a chemically caused condition where the cells of your body are in an "irritated mood." Within the lining of your blood vessels, this inflamed or aggravated state causes a response to abrasive injury that is an overreaction of sorts. (When you're in a bad mood, don't you overreact to small insults as well?) This excessive inflammation within your blood-vessel walls results in vascular and heart disease.

It is also well accepted that numerous degenerative diseases are inflammatory in nature, such as arthritis (joints), gastritis (stomach), Crohn's disease, diverticulitis, and ulcerative colitis (intestines), appendicitis, cancer, cirrhosis (liver), and diabetes. According to researcher Michèle Guerre-Millo,

> Our understanding of the relation between obesity and metabolic risk factors is growing rapidly. This understanding is based on the discovery of multiple products released from adipocytes [fat cells]. In the presence of obesity, these products are released in abnormal amounts. Each of these products has been implicated in the causation of one or another of the metabolic risk factors [above].[6]

High amounts of circulating fat molecules also cause your liver to respond by releasing harmful hormones into your body. In other words, a body in a "fat state" releases bad chemicals into your bloodstream, which wreak havoc on your anatomy! The take-home message? Lose the fat.

How do you know if you have metabolic syndrome? All you need is a tape measure, a blood-pressure cuff, and a few blood tests done after fasting. Clinically, the diagnosis is given to patients who demonstrate three or more of these factors:

1. Increased waist circumference (over 40 inches in men and over 35 inches in women)

2. Elevated triglycerides (150 mg/dl or higher)

3. Reduced HDL cholesterol (less than 40 mg/dl in men and less than 50 mg/dl in women)

4. Elevated blood pressure (130/85 or greater mmHg

5. Elevated glucose (100 mg/dl or higher)

Heed the Signs

As a physical therapist, I have been treating patients in outpatient orthopedic settings for over 20 years now. I can't tell you how many times this scenario occurs during an evaluation:

Mr. Jones, do you personally have any history of cardiovascular or heart disease?

No, I don't.

Do you have high blood pressure?

Not since I've been taking my medication.

Have you ever been told you have high cholesterol?

Yes, but the doctor says we'll just keep an eye on it…

How is your triglycerides level?

My what?

You don't have to have had a heart attack or be wearing a pacemaker in order to have heart disease. Markers (or signs) that you *presently* have heart and vascular problems are high blood pressure, high cholesterol (especially when your good vs. bad cholesterol ratio is poor), and high levels of circulating triglycerides. Another thing you should know is that many of the medications you take do not *cure* your body of cardiovascular disease. You still have cardiovascular disease, but the symptoms are being somewhat controlled.*

---

* Statins (Levacor, Zocor, Pravachol, Lipitor, Crestor), which are prescribed to lower cholesterol levels, have also been shown to reverse plaquing—cholesterol clots—within your blood-vessel walls. However, this "cure" comes at a high price. Not only does long-term medication usage adversely affect your liver, but statins can also cause muscle pain and weakness—both of which have ties to their depleting effect on the body's levels of CoQ10, an enzyme that is important in cellular respiration. Recently statins have been under investigation amid concerns that they may increase the risk of Parkinson's disease.[7]

Metabolic syndrome is very dangerous. If you are overweight or obese, please go to your primary care physician right away and have them give you a thorough exam, which should include *fasting* blood work. (This requires that you not eat or drink anything besides water for 12 hours before the blood draw.) You *need* to know how close to the edge you are with your health risks.

Joint Deterioration

Another obesity-related health problem is the physical pain and disability caused by premature structural breakdown of your weight-bearing joints. The joints most frequently affected in the overweight to obese patients I treat are those in their lower (lumbar) spine, as well as those in their hips, knees, ankles, and feet.

A quick description: A joint is the moving junction point or intersection between the ends of two bones. Typical joints have a fluid-filled capsule that surrounds the bones' ends (similar to vitamin E capsules). Within the joint capsules, the bone ends are surfaced with a glossy material called *cartilage*, which is perfectly designed to cushion the forces the joint must withstand as well as to provide the smooth gliding mechanism that must also exist within the joint.

Osteoarthritis is a disease process characterized by inflammation, breakdown, and eventual loss of this surface cartilage within the joints. Painful weight-bearing joints can create a significant loss of function…the worst part of which is the inability to walk for any significant distance without suffering a lot of pain. The simple fact is, your joints were created to bear a *normal* weight load, and that's the reason they tend to break down prematurely under an *excessive* load.

Good news, however. Even a 10 percent reduction in your body weight will have a considerable impact, reducing the pain from years of "joint overload." Overall, however, I must say I have had little lasting clinical success with my obese patients who come in with hip, knee, foot, or ankle pain that is the result of arthritis. There is only so much a therapist can do when joints are abused all day long, carrying a load they were never created to bear. This is another critical health risk to note down and consider.

Cancers

The diagnosis of cancer is enough to send fear-shivers down anyone's spine. As I mentioned before, fat (adipose) tissue releases hormones into the body that trigger an inflammatory response. Cancer, being inflammatory in nature, can be "egged on" by excess fat accumulation. In fact, numerous studies have shown that certain cancers thrive and multiply readily in a "fat" environment. These fat-loving cancers are, specifically, those of the *breast*, the *colon* (lower intestine), and *endometrial uterine* cancers. While endometrial cancer affects only women, breast and colon cancer can affect both men and women.

According to a recent study in the *New England Journal of Medicine*, there is an undeniable link between obesity and increased risk of death from *all* cancers. Study participants who had a BMI (body-mass index) of at least 40 (see chapter 2) had death rates from all cancers combined that were *52 percent higher* for men and *62 percent higher* for women than the rates found in men and women of normal weight.[8] It's downright undeniable—fat can cost you your life.

According to the National Cancer Institute (NCI), it's estimated that about 185,000 new cases of breast cancer will be diagnosed in the United States in 2008! And breast cancer will have claimed the lives of approximately 41,000 people by that same year's end. Further, the NCI estimates that another 108,000 people—mothers, sons, fathers, grandmothers—will be newly diagnosed with colon cancer in 2008. Over this same time period, the NCI also estimates that another 40,000 women will develop endometrial cancer, and 7000 of them will have lost the fight.

As high as these disease and death rates are, it is heartening to realize they could be dramatically reduced if people in the U.S. would return to their God-designed weight. Men, you could reduce your death rate from cancer by 52 percent. Women, your risk could drop by 62 percent. That's something worth working toward!

Why continue with a lifestyle that adds to your risk of developing such a feared disease and possibly even losing your life to it? Set your mind on restoring your body weight to the healthy range, and drop your odds of succumbing to this group of fat-loving cancers.

Obstructive Sleep Apnea

This sleep problem has been gaining more publicity as of late, so it's likely many of you may be familiar with it. *Sleep apnea* is by definition a condition in which breathing stops for more than 10 seconds during sleep. A person suffering from sleep apnea has frequent episodes (sometimes 400 to 500 per night) in which he or she stops breathing. Living well requires breathing well, but obesity is a major cause of this obstructive breathing problem, which has many harmful effects on your health.

According to the Mayo Clinic, the sudden drops in blood-oxygen levels that occur during sleep apnea increase your blood pressure and put undue strain on your cardiovascular system. Your risk of high blood pressure (hypertension) can be up to two to three times greater than if you sleep normally. The more severe your sleep apnea is (the greater the number of nonbreathing episodes per night), the greater your risk of high blood pressure. If there is underlying heart disease present, these multiple episodes of low blood oxygen (*hypoxia* or *hypoxemia*) can lead to sudden death from a heart attack. Obstructive sleep apnea also increases your risk of stroke *twofold to threefold*, regardless of whether or not you have high blood pressure.[9]

Many people are completely unaware that they suffer from this problem. Sure, they've been told they snore loudly or make funny noises as they sleep—but not breathing? That detail has escaped them. But these frequent arousals and the inability to achieve or maintain the deeper stages of restorative sleep can lead to excessive daytime sleepiness (with a tendency to quickly drop off to sleep during a quiet moment of the day when you're inactive), increased frequency of automobile accidents (drowsy driver), personality changes, decreased memory, erectile dysfunction (impotence), and depression.

How can you know whether *you* have obstructive sleep apnea? First of all, you are at greater statistical risk if you are an overweight male who is over 40 years old. In addition to the conditions listed in the previous paragraph, other common signs and symptoms are loud snoring, and frequent pauses during snoring that may be followed by choking or gasping. However, the only way to get an accurate diagnosis, complete with the number of breathing halts per night (which shows the severity of the problem), is to go to a sleep center and have a sleep study done. It takes only one night away from your life. Yet proper diagnosis and treatment of your sleep apnea could easily *add* many more nights back to your life! And I much prefer those odds.

Dementia

Dementia, usually thought to affect only the very aged, is a progressive disease of the brain characterized by the slow loss of memory. The first brain function to be lost is the short-term memory, followed eventually by long-term memory loss. Advanced states of dementia leave the affected person unable to recognize even their loved ones. Dementia steals away the person, yet leaves their body.

I bet you never even thought your overweight or obese state would have an effect on your brain, but it most certainly does! Your brain's health is dependent upon two basic needs: glucose (sugar molecules) and oxygen. Though sugar deficits are not the problem here, by having a BMI and waist circumference greater than normal, you've likely set up two previously discussed conditions that are decreasing oxygen flow to your brain: cardiovascular disease and obstructive sleep apnea. By narrowing your blood vessels, cardiovascular disease decreases the overall blood flow to your brain. The less blood flow, the less available oxygen. Sleep apnea decreases brain oxygen levels simply because oxygen that doesn't get drawn into your lungs will not get to your brain!

Next to dying from cancer, most people declare that their biggest health fear for the future is that of "losing their mind"—even beyond being physically disabled. Watching my mother suffer with dementia while having full function of her physical body, I have to say I agree with this. For the person suffering with it, a wasting mind is worse than a wasting body—and this is also the case for the loved ones who must endure the process along with the sufferer. It is not too late for you. You have the power to affect the aging process of your brain by changing your food intake. Purpose to be helpful and useful to yourself and to those who love you. A mind is a terrible thing to waste.

Other Disease Risks

Sadly, there's more that can be brought on by overweight and obesity, such as

- gallbladder disease (cholesterol gallstones)
- fatty liver disease (where healthy liver tissue is replaced with fat, which is often a precursor to liver cancer)
- abdominal hernias (from the internal pressure of excess fat)
- varicose veins
- gout

Each and every one of these diseases has been shown to be highly correlated with obesity.

⟞⟝

I realize this chapter has become overwhelmingly sad. Yet it was my intention from the beginning to get your attention. I wanted you to see an undeniable—and motivating—list of significant costs you've been enduring because of your problems with food.

But there is an exit door, a way out from the place you've been trapped in—before the next social, occupational, or bodily disease barges in, threatening your life or at least your emotional stability. In the following chapter we'll examine many reasons people are driven to overeat. I believe you'll identify with at least one of them. No cure has ever come without a proper diagnosis, so once you positively grasp *why* you do what you do, you can begin the journey toward healing and recovery—recovery for a *lifetime*.

Kelly's Story of Hope

I have battled with being overweight for most of my life. My growing-up years were very unstable—my family moved nearly a dozen times. My mother and father fought often, usually over my dad's many adulterous affairs. My father ran our home using intimidation tactics. He made our mealtimes something to be dreaded. Because I was overweight, he ridiculed me daily with name-calling, and he used to force me to drink water mixed with vinegar before every meal to fill my stomach so I wouldn't "eat so much."

After I'd lived 17 years under such oppressive control, my father died quite suddenly from liver cancer. My mother quickly took on a boyfriend, and I was left to parent myself. I remember feeling very disoriented. So in addition to my food addiction, I began using marijuana—which only intensified my hunger!

My struggle with weight continued as I grew older. I became a Christian at 24 years old and continued not to deal with the whole weight issue. Even as I grew in my understanding and relationship with the Lord, I never looked at my overeating from a spiritual perspective. I viewed it purely as a lack of self-control.

Fast-forward many years…life for me became more difficult. While my husband and I were dealing with years of infertility, desperately yearning for a child of our own, my mother passed away. Truthfully, at that point, I was making every excuse for overindulging in food. As a result of using food for pain relief, I saw my weight balloon up to 250 pounds! It was during a routine doctor's visit in 2000 that I learned that my blood pressure was so high that it required me to go on medication.

⁕

Six years later, in April 2006, I remember not feeling quite right. At a routine visit with my gynecologist, my blood-sugar test showed that my level was up over 200 (that's twice as high as normal!). When the nurse took my blood pressure, it was very high as well. I was told to see my regular doctor immediately. I was scared, so I did exactly what I was told.

At my regular doctor's office my blood-sugar level tested at 280! I was told, quite frankly, that I had full-blown diabetes. My doctor ordered further blood work, which showed that my bad cholesterol was over 200 and my good cholesterol was not high enough. Also included in my blood work was a hemoglobin A1c blood test, which shows the average of your sugar levels over the past three months. It came back as a 9, when normal is below 6. I was now told I had to take three medications, one for my high blood pressure, one for my cholesterol, and one for my diabetes. I went from being scared to being terrified! My doctor put me on a strict diet and said to come back in a month.

One week later, while I was at a Wednesday-night class at my church, I asked a friend to pray for me. She told me she was thinking about starting a Christ-centered weight loss program. I was beyond interested—talk about God's timing! We agreed to begin in the next few weeks.

The eating plan my doctor gave me started getting easier, and through the accompanying weight-loss Bible study, God was showing me how I was clearly going against His will with what I was doing to myself. Even with my little bit of obedience, He was changing me; making me healthier!

I went back to the doctor. After only a month my sugar was already coming down. My blood pressure was decreasing as well. And my bad cholesterol had dropped to 167, low enough, my doctor said, so that I could come off that medicine. I was told to once again come back in a month.

When my next appointment came, I had lost more than 20 pounds. My blood pressure had come down so much that he started weaning me off of that medicine as well! My sugar level was down to 108! My doctor asked me to come back in a month's time so he could recheck my blood pressure. That next month my pressure was normal, and he told me to go off the medicine all together.

⚜

Through this time of recovery, God has shown me His mercy and love for me. I now realize that He cares about what I put in my mouth. He loves me so much and does not want me to damage the body He's given me. He showed me that the food was just a fleeting enjoyment, but a healthy body was so much more.

Today I am down 75 pounds from my heaviest point. At my last doctor's visit my blood pressure was 90/60 and my fasting sugar level was 90 with a new hemoglobin A1c result of 6.5. My doctor laughed as he asked me where the rest of me went! I was pronounced to no longer have high blood pressure or diabetes—I was perfectly healthy.

It has been three years since my health crisis. I have kept most of the weight off, but have struggled a bit. I know I need to press on and always be aware of the connection between my emotions and my eating.

I wish I could have avoided that health scare, but I now thank God for that wake-up call. God will always bless our good choices in life. I picture Him just waiting there to cheer on my obedience. I still have days of struggle, battling my desire to use food for comfort. But I look how far God has led me, and that makes it easier to say no to overeating. He will continue to help me in every struggle I have—all I need to do is ask! He wants to be my comfort during the rough times. I am working on letting Him do just that. I am a work in progress.

Don't you know that your body is a temple of the Holy Spirit, who is in you, whom you have received from God? You are not your own, you were bought at a price. Therefore honor God with your body.

1 Corinthians 6:19-20

Chapter 3

Why You Binge

Tell yourself the truth.

I *just love food!"*
Don't many people say this to try to convince others—and themselves—that they don't have a problem? They don't *abuse* food; they simply *enjoy* its taste. The alternative, that they're using food to fulfill an unaddressed need, is something they aren't ready or willing to face. (Better to remain a food lover than a food addict.)

In reality, there are a great number of possible reasons why you eat more food than what your body requires to live. And loving the taste of food, while certainly a valid reason, doesn't always correlate with being overweight. According to Jane Jakubczak, a registered dietician who runs a weight-loss clinic at the University of Maryland, "75 percent of overeating is caused by emotions." Everyone eats for emotional reasons at one time or another. For you, however, this emotional eating has likely become chronic. Would you be willing to peer over the top of the wall you've been barricading your emotions behind and consider what is perhaps *your* psychological reason or reasons for overeating?

What Makes Comfort Food So Very Comforting?

I love how, given time, money, and research, so many of life's questions get answered. I guess I'm just a bit of a science junkie, because it thrills me when science provides explanations for how things were designed by our Creator to function. Take the well-known and accepted "comfort foods"—fried chicken, cheeseburgers, french fries, potato chips, mashed potatoes, chocolate…They are the go-to foods when you are stressed out, overtired, and overworked. Why? What makes these food so very satisfying?

It has been discovered that certain foods change the chemistry of your brain. Chemicals such as *cannabinoids* and *serotonin* are produced after you eat the comfort foods. Now, does that word *cannabinoids* ring a bell with anyone? Any reformed pot smokers? The scientific name for the plant from which the street drug pot (weed, marijuana) comes is *cannabis*. You may be surprised to know that the compounds that are released into your brain when you eat fried or high-fat foods are from the same family of chemicals released when people smoke a joint of marijuana. Both the plant-based and the food-based sources give you a temporary emotional or mental high.

Why does your brain like this chemical so much? In answer, here's an illustration: Consider each of your responsibilities and worries to be contained in its own separate file. Your brain then stacks all those files in an orderly pile. At the top of the pile are your most worrisome folders—at the bottom, your least. Enter a flood of cannabinoids. It is as if a hoodlum enters your file room and, just for fun, knocks your neatly stacked folder pile to the floor. He proceeds to scatter the files about so that the ones that were weighing most heavily on your mind are no longer on the top of the pile, staring you down. The result in your brain? *"No worries, mon!"* (This is a phrase I picked up during my vacation to the island of Jamaica—regardless of my request, the hotel staff would respond with this friendly, reassuring saying.)

Foods such as chocolate that make more serotonin available have a soothing effect on your mind, as serotonin is a "happy" brain chemical. Too little of it is associated with depression. In fact, most medications prescribed to combat depression alter the brain's ability to accept or produce more serotonin. (Comedian Anita Renfroe does a piece called "The Four *Mood* Groups": chocolate, cheese, french fries, and potato chips. It's hilarious. You see, you and I—and Anita—know it instinctively: Certain foods just *feel* better than others!)

Food—It's Here, There, and Everywhere!

We live under a daily bombardment of food advertisements—on TV, in magazines, on the radio, online, on billboards along the highway. They are simply unavoidable. If you are hungry, these ads will lure you toward a food vendor, who next places a scrumptious-looking image in front of you or makes the suggestion that you can "have it your way." And even when you're not hungry—not even thinking about food—the mere mention, sight, or even aroma of one of these food establishments can start your mouth watering and your gastric juices flowing. Who hasn't been tempted as they walk past a Cinnabon store in the mall?

Now swing the pendulum the other way. What is the media reminding you of every single day? That you are beautiful only if you are thin and appear perfect. I have been told that photographers, thanks to the ease of digital manipulation, regularly slim the hips and enlarge the bustlines of their female subjects; male actors and models have their "love handles" trimmed down with a few clicks of the computer's mouse. And we consumers are left feeling like we will *never* measure up, no matter how much weight we lose or muscle mass we gain. So why even bother? When a goal is that unattainable, why try? These conflicting messages are enough to make someone a bipolar food consumer: *eat, eat, eat...no...diet, diet, diet!*

In most societies food equals celebration and refreshment, which, in moderation, is appropriate. I truly believe that God created food to enjoy and to bring us satisfaction—or He wouldn't have gone to the trouble to create the tiny taste buds that line our tongues. And eating is refreshing...if we are depleted. But we have far crossed the line. We celebrate *everything* with food. Each time a child completes something (fifth grade, soccer season, school concert) we tend to celebrate with a food party. Every company success is drowned in a sea of submarine sandwiches and potato salad. And if your church is anything like mine, all events conclude with a refined-carbohydrate-and-sugar buffet table.

Joyce Meyer, a popular Christian speaker, shared a quip in her book *Eat Well, Stay Thin.* She said that in the Bible, the apostle Paul wrote that he daily "buffets" his body—which, when pronounced "BUFF-it," would mean he trains or disciplines his body. Meyers said that, rather, too many Christians "buff-AY" their bodies, gorging upon whatever is in front of them. To that I say, *Amen, sister!* But it doesn't have to be that way.

Nothin' to Do...

This is one reason for overeating we almost all have in common: boredom. Who hasn't sat on the couch or at a party you really didn't feel like being at, and picked up a handful of chips and started in on them? Problem is, once you start you just keep on eating until it's time to go to bed, it's time to leave, or the food runs out.

What exactly is boredom? It is by definition 1) lack of interest in a redundant task, 2) an inability to change an uninteresting situation, or 3) an inability to engage oneself with the world around. I want to emphasize the last reason for boredom because it looks an awful lot like depression to me. In fact, boredom and depression are highly related, according to the literature. If you find yourself feeling bored much of the time, consider that what you may be feeling is actually a form of *depression*. If this is the case, you're using food as a mood elevator. In other words, when your life feels empty, you fill your stomach instead.

Gotta Have It Now!

Today, delayed gratification is in short supply. The idea of working toward something and having to wait for a reward is foreign to many. In the generation or so since the microwave arrived, we have become a "gotta have it now" people. Parents quickly give in to their children's whims and whines (often feeding them to keep them quiet). As a result, young ones are raised without an ability to delay gratification, which makes it difficult for them to live disciplined lives once they reach adulthood. The inability to delay gratification is a major reason for the nation's mortgage crisis and fiscal indebtedness, for impulsiveness in classrooms, in boardrooms, and on the roadways, for sexual promiscuity (followed by epidemic venereal disease rates) and—the subject we are discussing in this book—our obesity epidemic.

Does this sound similar to the way you were raised? You may be feeling the effects of your childhood beginning to show themselves in your food consumption. When you see something you want to eat or drink you absolutely must have it. You want not just one bite, you want the whole thing! Let me say, though, that it is possible to retrain yourself to wait, to limit, and to sometimes completely abstain from feeding yourself. That's the purpose of this book.

Out of Control

Growing up, maybe you had to endure a life where everything seemed out of control—finances, relationships, the mental stability of your caregivers, the order within your home. (I know this type of upbringing quite well.) Or perhaps the opposite was true. You were raised by an inflexible, controlling parent. As with most extremes, neither of these situations is an atmosphere in which people *thrive*. Rather, they create a basic-instinct need to *survive*.

So how might a small child respond to home-life stress from "out-of-control" or "overcontrol"? Enter the most basic of human experiences—eating. There are not many things a child can take charge of in an "out of *their* control" environment. But food intake and "output"—now that is something they can be master over!

What happens to these troubled kids? Well, for one thing, they grow up. But when these grown up, food-misusing people take their place in adult society, they struggle to gain control over the very thing they thought was giving them control in the first place. Over the years, I have witnessed very sad polar-opposite outcomes among some of the patients I've treated. Some of my patients who lived "out of *their* control" childhoods became anorexic. Conversely, some became overusers of food, which resulted in bingeing and purging, or simply bingeing.

A few years back, one of my patients, a 16-year-old girl, readily admitted to me that she had a problem with anorexia. In fact, she had to be hospitalized before she gained freedom from its stranglehold. If you are working through this book, you are probably not withholding food from yourself. However, in either situation, I want you to be fully aware that both extremes of food control will end in premature death, though one may arrive sooner than the other.

The topic of "output" is also part of this control issue. From time to time pediatricians have to deal with children who are preventing themselves from having a bowel movement. Children can cause themselves to become so extremely constipated that their pediatrician must tell the parent to begin adding mineral oil to their baby bottles or sippy cups. Many of these constipation cases are psychologically caused. These children are simply seeking to have control over *something*!

As people age, they realize the physical pain involved in "backing up their plumbing," so for some, output control takes the form of vomiting after meals. This condition, as you likely know, is called *bulimia*. Others turn to laxatives in hope of quickly flushing all those calories from their bodies before they have a chance to land somewhere in their midsections. Food, however, is meant for nourishment, and what goes down someone's throat is meant to come naturally out the other end. Manipulating this process in any way points to a life in need of help. As an adult who is seeking a new relationship with food, you are in the position to begin taking back control over your life—this time in a healthy way. Food no longer has to control you.

In Dire Need of a Tranquilizer

Life can be full of painful circumstances—and for some people there seems to be an unfair amount. I've always felt I had to endure more than my fair share of childhood hardships and emotional pain. Yet when I look around, there are always others who have had to endure more. But truthfully, life's emotional hardships are not a contest to be won or lost based on who's had more. Whatever *you* have had to endure has been or still is painful for *you*!

Each of us has had to find a way to survive the pain. If the coping mechanism you've chosen is healthy, your "survive" turns into "thrive." But if you've chosen to deal with your emotional pain with food, then you are a food addict…just like a person who pops tranquilizers is a drug addict. You are attempting to numb your pain with food. Without honestly naming your reason or reasons for overeating, you will never—*never*—be released from its bondage. And I would love to see you walk in freedom.

"I Can't Right Now…I'm Eating"

We are so clever at avoiding things we don't want to do or situations we don't want to deal with. Do you have a mountain of laundry staring you in the face? Is there a difficult phone call you're supposed to make? Is the lawn ten days overgrown and still growing? And how about all those cluttered, booby-trap closets around your house? One false move and their contents will come tumbling down. You know you should get to the task, but wait just a minute…or 30…you just heard the refrigerator calling you. Or was it the pantry? Eating to avoid dealing with a problem or situation is food abuse. You are handling food—*handing* yourself food—instead of handling your responsibilities.

Stressed Out!

So many people today live with their life's glass of water poured way too high. All it takes is one more thing added to your glass—your life—and water spills over the edge. Or rather, you have a meltdown: a fit of rage, a crying fest, a pity fest. Each meltdown of course ends in an eating fest!

I have a friend who is fully aware that she overeats when she's had to endure a high-pressure day. Yet without another way to deal with her stress, she must constantly return to her "tried-and-true" method. Stress makes you so unhappy that in order to restore your balance you fill yourself with temporary happiness in the form of chemical pleasure. (Recall our discussion on the chemical nature of comfort foods!) Instead of using a healthy stress release such as exercise, talking to a trusted person, or taking part in a recreational or creative activity, you eat. It's quick, it's available, and it's easy. But it's *not* free.

Anger and Depression

I'm not sure if you've ever thought of it this way, but anger and depression are close cousins—in fact, they're more like brothers. You see, anger is a volatile emotion that is usually expressed outwardly (though many seethe internally with it). Depression is the emotion of anger turned inward. I have never met a person who battles depression who isn't angry about something—whether or not they're conscious of it.

Interestingly, a study was performed in which chronically angry people were found to consume about *600 more calories per day* than people who were not angry by nature.[1] Food temporarily soothes the angry beast within. Yet as a result of bingeing, you now add a new object of anger—yourself. You're angry that you've overeaten. You're angry over your lack of self-control. You may even be feeling physically uncomfortable or sick from the food you just gorged on, so you're angry that you've caused yourself discomfort. You will need to realize that anger management and resolution cannot include food.

Protection from Sexual Intimacy

Scientific studies show that 20 to 30 percent of heterosexuals who suffer with obesity have a self-reported history of sexual abuse.[2] Furthermore, in 2007 *Obesity*, a research journal, reported that 39 percent of obese lesbian women have an admitted history of sexual abuse. Only 25 percent of non-obese lesbians report such a history.[3] (I wonder how many of the research participants were not able to admit their history.) This study clearly exposes the relationship between obesity and childhood sexual abuse. Though it doesn't offer any insight into the overweight but not obese population, it seems likely that we'd find sexual abuse to be prevalent there as well.

Many innocent people have been made to associate their physical bodies with someone else's sexual sin—and with shame. If this abhorrent abuse is part of your personal background, you may be subconsciously trying to protect yourself from any further violation, or any sexual attention for that matter, by building a fence around yourself. Society has told you that others aren't sexually attracted to fat people. So fat you became—simply to protect yourself against anyone's sexual advances.

Oh, sweet soul, your sexuality was made to be enjoyed *within God's plan for it.* In the next few chapters you will see how you can be restored and made pure again. Yes, *pure.* Sexual purity can be regained by the renewing of your mind and your emotions. (More on this subject in chapters 6 and 8.) But for now, don't continue assaulting your body, exchanging past sexual abuse by another for present physical abuse by food at your own hands.

Who, Me?

Denial. Some of you may be living your life day to day, bingeing on food and avoiding looking into any mirrors, especially when undressed. You deny the extent of your weight problem, you deny the risks to your health and the effect on your relationships and work situation, and you deny that you are out of control with food. When you get out of breath climbing up a few steps, you tell yourself you are "just out of shape."

Maybe the only reason you're reading this book is because someone who cares for you has "run an intervention." They've said, "Please, read this book—I love you and I don't want to lose you." So even though you don't understand what the concern is about, you agreed to read it. For you, I simply ask that you continue with an open mind and an open heart…this book was written with you in mind.

At a Loss for Love…

In our culture, the heart has always been the holder for our emotions. We love people "with all our heart" or we can hide hatred within our "heart." I once heard a missionary describe his experience translating the concept of "inviting Jesus into your heart" for a remote tribal village. In these people's language, the *throat* was the center of all things, so the gospel message had to be described as accepting the gift of salvation offered by Jesus by inviting Him to live in their throats! Wherever we view our emotions as stored, we were created with a deep-seated need to feel loved, be loved, and express love.

In his book *The Five Love Languages*, author Gary Chapman says that love can be offered and received in five distinct ways: through quality time, words of affirmation, acts of service, touch (nonsexual), and gifts. Chapman believes that each person has a primary way in which they receive love (and usually they extend love in the same manner). He proposes that some people may *feel* unloved not because they weren't loved as they were raised, but because their love language was not "spoken" to them. Take that into the present. Many of you may not feel loved because no one in your life is speaking your particular love language to you.

Some of you, sadly, had *no* love language spoken to you. You were called a problem, a mistake, a pain-in-the-you-know-what, and much worse. You may have been physically, emotionally, or sexually abused. Whichever it was, it was made crystal clear to you that you were not worthy of being properly loved.

I must denounce that untruth here and now. You are worthy of being loved. You are lovable. You deserve to be loved. Listen carefully: Hurt people hurt people. Wounded people wound people. Broken people try to break people. Don't allow another person's brokenness to ruin your future—even if they soiled your past. Seek healing. Chapter 7 will show you how to achieve this by filling your heart instead of your stomach.

⌘

Though this chapter is certainly not 100 percent complete, I believe every one of you who has been honestly assessing the material has identified at least one reason—possibly three or four—as *your* reason or reasons for overeating. If it seems to you that none of the issues I've discussed are *your* issues, let me suggest that you ask someone who knows you well to give their input. (If you are sincerely seeking the truth, let them speak in all honesty.) Be open to the fact that the pain from your past may have created a blind spot that is now hindering your self-assessment.

In the following chapter we will take an honest look at the problem of out-of-control eating. And let's now call it what it probably is: *food addiction*. We'll consider the course addiction runs when left to itself, and the two ways you can break free from this vicious cycle. In chapter 5 we will delve deeper into the primary emotions underlying your abuse of food. Then in chapters 6 through 10 you will find effective approaches that will enable you to climb up out of your emotional pit and break the cycle of addiction for good!

Chapter 4

The Not-So-Merry-Go-Round of Food Addiction

Negative emotions fuel your food-addiction cycle.

M any things in nature were created to function in a cycle, a series of revolving, sequenced, predictable happenings. The participant in a cycle is subject to an intrinsic driving force to "complete the loop." Consider the life cycle of a butterfly. Worm one day, cocoon another—and then a beautiful butterfly emerges. Eggs are laid, worms hatch, then more cocoons, followed by more butterflies. A tree will grow, produce leaves, and those leaves eventually fall to the ground. Predictably, those fallen leaves decompose into soil, which then serves to nourish the roots of that very same plant. In this way the plant completes its determined cycle and continues to grow. These two examples of beneficial, God-designed cyclical processes, which exist to benefit the "participant," are often referred to as *life cycles*.

Some cycles, however, offer no benefit at all. In fact, they have toxic effects on whatever is held captive in their loops. We might even refer to them as *death cycles*. In nature we don't have to look far in order to find examples. Take modern farming, for instance. By using pesticides to protect our crops, we have inadvertently killed off many of the honeybee populations that pollinate the flowers of our fruit trees and produce. Fewer bees mean less pollination, and without adequate pollination, we have a reduction in the amount of fruit and vegetables produced. So in order to "safeguard" our declining crops, we use more pesticides...which in turn kills more bees. We can also find examples

63

of negative cycles within everyday society, such as welfare, national debt, fatherless children, and drug and alcohol dependency.

While each negative cycle is unique in its stages, all are similar in this: with human beings, they create a pervasive sense of helplessness for whoever is stuck in them. Those riding on one of these not-so-merry-go-rounds experience a sense of *Why bother? Things (or I) will never change. I could never live a different life.* If you're on such a ride, you likely feel powerless to get off. All you can do is just hang on for the rest of the miserable trip—which you are certain will end badly.

⊸◊⊶

No matter how you choose to look at it, food addiction qualifies as a negative, destructive cycle, or as I called it earlier, a "death cycle." Maybe you've never thought about your eating problem in terms of a cycle before—nor an addiction! The dictionary defines *addiction* as

> The state of being enslaved to a habit or practice or to something that is psychologically or physically habit-forming.

According to this definition, *food addiction* can be defined as:

> Being unable to break free from the habit of eating too much because you mentally, emotionally, or physically can't seem to live (cope) without it.

Does this sounds a lot like what you're dealing with?

What exactly does this food-addiction cycle look like? If you study the diagram below, you'll note that there are six distinct stages in this death cycle.

The Unbroken Cycle of Food Addiction

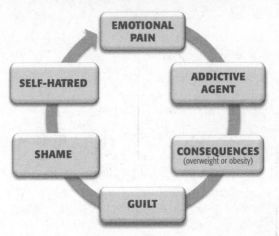

Beginning at the top of the circle, *emotional pain* is the first "horse" on this not-so-merry-go-round. Following the diagram around clockwise, the food addict chooses food as his *addictive agent*—as a means of dealing with this pain in the heart. Overeating, though bringing temporary pain relief, yields long-term *consequences* (overweight/obesity, disease, and so on—see chapter 2). When an overeater looks in the mirror, steps on the bathroom scale, or even looks at the empty packaging of what they've just consumed, *guilt* rushes in like a flood. Guilt is quickly followed by two even stronger "natural disasters," the hurricane of *shame* and the tornado of *self-hatred*. Once you've allowed yourself to ride completely around this not-so-merry-go-round, you've done nothing but add to your original load of emotional pain.

All addictions must have two "participants": the *addict* and the *addictive agent*. In alcoholism, you have the alcoholic and his booze. In drug addiction you have the junkie and his dope. Now…if you are the "eater" in the food-addiction cycle, then *you,* my friend, are the addict. And your addictive agent is food.

There are two telltale signs that mark any addiction—1) the addict is simply unable to stop themselves from overindulging, and 2) the cycle they are engaged in is harming their life.

Addictions typically continue until one of three things happens:

1. The addict hits "rock bottom."
2. A concerned onlooker runs some kind of an "intervention."
3. Sorrowfully, the addiction takes the life of the addict (the death cycle is completed).

Are You a Food Addict?

The word *addict* often brings to mind an unkempt person staggering down the sidewalk, clearly under the influence of some mind-altering substance. Would you be willing to lay aside such unpleasant images for a moment and seriously ask yourself a few questions? According to Dr. David Hawkins in his book *Breaking Everyday Addictions,* the indications of addiction are found in honest answers to a few deep questions.[1]

1. Do you have a compulsive physical or psychological dependence, or both, on food?
2. Do you continue to overeat in spite of obvious consequences?
3. Do you continue to eat beyond the "full feeling"?
4. Do you lie about how much you eat, deny your overeating problem, or even hide the "evidence" when you've eaten?
5. Have you allowed your life (weight) to become unmanageable?

If you find yourself answering yes to most or all of these questions, then you've arrived at your answer...you are indeed addicted to food.

Hitting rock bottom in food addiction could take the form of reaching a new high weight point; it could be receiving the diagnosis of a very serious weight-related disease. Maybe your rock bottom will be that you're fed up with yourself and can't stand another day lived in this addiction! As for an intervention, I hope you will allow this book to be just that. It is my sincere desire to help you change your life's course in regard to overeating. You may be reading this book because someone else in your life has intervened, saying, "I can't bear the thought of losing you prematurely. It's time for you to get control over your weight!" As for the third way this cycle could end, premature death, I pray you will never know this ending.

The Hungry Heart

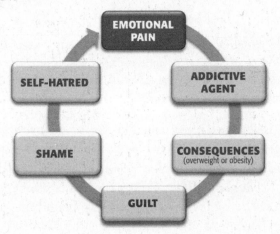

Food addiction typically begins with emotional pain or emotional hunger. Food can be an addictive agent in an attempt to numb or mask the heart's pain. Research has confirmed that in many cases the root of this pain is abuse. When I say *abuse*, what thoughts come to your mind? Sexual, physical, or verbal abuse? These obvious forms are known by psychologists as *active abuse*. Also included in this category is emotional violence (manipulation) or a rigid, overcontrolled living environment. These forms of abuse are usually easy to spot, easy to label, and hard to deny.

Yet there's a more subtle type of abuse that you may have endured (as did I), which you've probably never thought of as actual *abuse*. Labeled *passive abuse* by the psychology community, this type is more difficult for the untrained eye to detect, yet it can be equally as damaging.

Passive abuse takes place when a child is *passively* raised or even ignored. Possibly you were in such a home—raised by distracted parents or caregivers. Some of you may have had a parent who was physically or mentally ill. Some of you had caregivers who were emotionally cold, so that you remained untouched by loving hands and uncaressed by tender words. Maybe your parents were preoccupied with their work, their household chores, or even their marital woes. Passive abuse is by omission, rather than commission. According to psychiatrists Frank Minirth and Paul Meier of the Minirth-Meier Clinic,

> To develop into healthy adults, children must receive time, attention and affection from their parents. If any of these qualities was missing or compromised in your family of origin, then there was passive abuse.[2]

If what is described here sounds like your home environment, then you'll likely agree that, since you weren't raised in an atmosphere where you could thrive, you had no other choice but to survive. The result of such a deficient upbringing leaves the passively abused child to wonder whether they have any value to their parents or family members. And since their home mirrors the world to them, they wonder if they have any value at all to anyone.

My Own Experience

Looking back on my own childhood, I can honestly say that my mother and father would not receive high marks on their parenting. They failed to provide a nurturing environment for the emotional stability of their children. Most of the "discipline" I underwent as a youngster was meted out in anger (which would make it punishment rather than discipline), and it would likely be called physical (active) abuse by today's standards. There was much verbal criticism and emotional manipulation.

Likewise, my upbringing was littered with passive abuse (emotional neglect). My father worked six days a week, and on the seventh day—well, let's just say every Sunday looked like this: Sunday school, church, then home for lunch and for my father to read three Sunday newspapers cover to cover, dinner, then finally back to church for the evening service. No amount of dancing around my father's reading chair or begging for him to play with me could get his attention. The only thing that caused him to glance toward me was when I got into mischief—typically by torturing my two younger brothers. I got his attention all right—negative attention, but attention nonetheless! That had to suffice.

My mother, on the other hand, was too busy keeping up with the housework or battling her often crippling depression to be much of a parent. In fact, I have no childhood memories of her ever playing with me or reading to me! When I was 11, she lost her sister to cancer. Because of her mental instability, my mother cried almost daily for what I remember to be nearly three years! I was forced, as a fifth-grader, to become the "parentified child" and had to mother my own mother from that point on—providing for her emotional nurturing. Sadly, my childhood memories are filled with thoughts of anger and insecurity rather than harmony and contentment.

So if, upon careful reflection on your own life, you can describe yourself as having experienced things you shouldn't have (active abuse), having lacked some of the essential elements of parenting (passive abuse), or both, then you, as I did, have grown up with an empty, hungry heart.

An Empty Heart

Most empty-heart syndromes begin in childhood, but you can certainly have your heart "emptied" in adulthood. Your emotional hunger may stem from a difficult marriage or an abusive spouse. Or maybe you've suffered some severe trauma, disappointment, or disease. Whether the initial source of your emotional pain came in childhood or adulthood, you must consider the likelihood that it has driven you to become a food addict. You have sought to fill your heart hunger with food.

Unfortunately, the problem with food addiction is, no matter how much you fill your stomach, your *heart* still remains empty! Your emotional pain persists. If thoughts of certain situations that have gone into creating your hungry heart are beginning to come to mind, jot them down in your notebook. (At this point a simple list will do. We'll take a more thorough approach in chapter 5.)

A Full Stomach

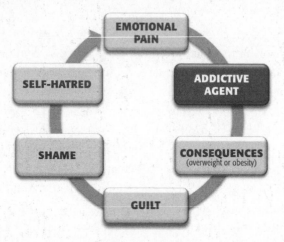

The second stage of the food-addiction cycle is overconsumption of your addictive agent: food. (And let's not forget drink for those of you who love milkshakes or soda pop.) Being driven to eat is like having an itchy mosquito bite. The more you scratch, the more you *have* to scratch. It only quits itching when you've finally scratched so hard that you've broken the skin, and now, instead of sending out "itchy" messages, all it tells you is that it's in pain!

Overeating is just that. You'll often find yourself eating until you almost feel sick (in pain). When will you learn to stop before you get so uncomfortable? Or better yet—when will you be able to stop before you even get started? You tell yourself, *If food just didn't taste so good—and if it wasn't so easy to come by...*Your trigger foods can call to you anytime, day or night! In the last chapter we talked about the scientific reasons behind food cravings. What is it you crave? Chocolate? French fries? Pasta? A Starbucks Mocha Frappuccino? As we've been talking about, what you crave goes far beyond what you put in your mouth. There will be more about that in chapter 7. But for right now, hold that thought as we continue to follow the progression of the food-addiction cycle.

The Consequences

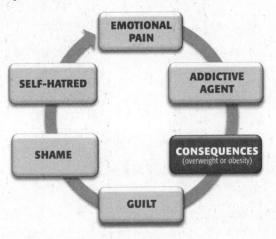

There are consequences to everything we do. In the case of an addiction, they're always bad. No one likes the aftermath of overeating—the bloating, the indigestion, the sluggishness...But what's worse is the continual increase in your size. When you gain a lot of weight, it's not just your clothes that don't fit. *Life* no longer seems to fit. As you've no doubt recognized, this world is not sized flexibly. You may have trouble getting into a theater chair or an airplane seat. When you're invited to someone's home for a meal, a narrow armchair can be an unwelcome sight. Recreational activities, such as rides at the amusement park, become something to be dreaded rather than enjoyed. In fact, most of the recreational activities you used to enjoy have had to fall by the wayside. Suffice it to say, the consequences of not fitting in lead to yet more emptiness and pain.

Guilty as Charged

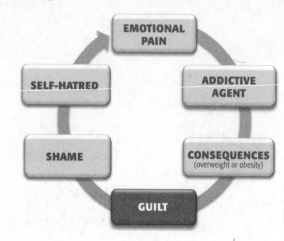

Guilt is a complex emotion. It can be a very real and accurate assessment of your situation. For example, if you steal something, lie, or deliberately hurt someone (even yourself, as is the case with overeating), remorse over your actions is an entirely appropriate response. You did something you know to be wrong or hurtful. You feel guilty, and that emotion is correct thinking, analyzed truthfully.

On the other hand, guilt can be an emotion that is falsely arrived at, or even handed to you by another (maybe as a "gift" from your mother!). In this case someone has suggested that your actions were inappropriate and that you should feel bad about them. It is an opinion rendered by another that has been erroneously taken on by you, the victim of secondhand guilt.

Authentic guilt is not necessarily bad, even though it may feel so at first. If it is managed constructively, truthful guilt can lead to personal growth through repentance and reform (more in chapter 6). However, if it is not dealt with and allowed to fester, guilt will prove to be destructive. It is undealt-with guilt that maintains the cycle of food addiction, leading you into further bondage.

Shame on You!

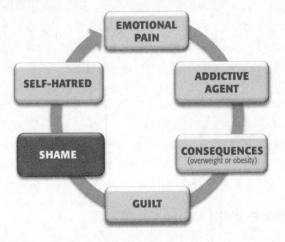

What exactly is the difference between guilt and shame? True guilt is a *fact* or *state* of having committed an offense or wrong that is accompanied by a *feeling* of responsibility or remorse. With overeating, guilt is a normal, healthy response to bingeing. Shame, on the other hand, is the punishing form of guilt. The shame portion of the food-addiction cycle is a negative judgment of yourself in your own mind's eye. Psychologist John Bradshaw says it well:

> Guilt says I've done something wrong; shame says there is something wrong with *me*. Guilt says I've made a mistake; shame says *I* am a mistake. Guilt says what I did was not good; shame says *I* am no good.[3]

Guilt is a feeling supported by a factual event, but shame is character assassination. It moves you beyond an incident and creates a negative generalization about your whole self. It makes you feel altogether, hopelessly embarrassed and unworthy. If emotional pain is the fuel behind your food-addiction cycle, then shame supercharges it, making sure you, its victim, stay locked into its downward-spiraling loop.

Some of you may have entered the addiction cycle already fueled with your own supply of shame. Can you remember anyone scolding you with these words: "You should be ashamed of yourself"? Shame can be shoved upon you under false pretenses, as the result of false guilt over something in which you had no control, such as being impoverished or having a physical disability. Maybe you suffer shame as the result of what is called *carried guilt*.[4] This is the guilt children will "carry on themselves," such as the condemning thoughts that their parents got divorced because they were bad kids, or taking responsibility for their parent being depressed all the time.

When the pain of all this past shame teams up with shame over being overweight or obese, you are in for one scary ride on the not-so-merry-go-round of food addiction.

Despising the Very Skin You're In

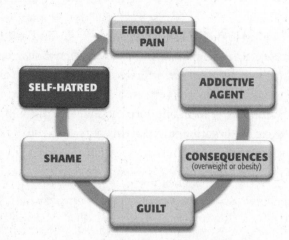

Self-hatred is the last stage before the "ride" begins all over again. It is barely distinguishable from shame at first glance. But if you were to pick up a magnifying glass and look at it, you'd see that it's hate mixed with disgust. Because shame leaves you feeling unworthy, disgraced, and deeply embarrassed, the next "logical" thought is to hate yourself. (Your parents were correct—*hate* is a strong word.) At this point of the cycle you confirm your self-disgust by not caring how much you weigh or what food addiction is costing you...because you are certain you don't deserve anything good, only punishment. So you become your own punisher. You abuse yourself because that's what you've determined you deserve. Deep in your subconscious you may even think, *Other people abused me, so that's all I'm worthy of—abuse.*

❧

If this is where you are today—trapped in this death cycle—my heart is weeping for you. You were created neither to be abused nor to abuse yourself. You were created to live in freedom and experience joy. Yes, painful experiences have occurred in your life. And yes, it's likely you will have to live through other situations that will cause you further emotional pain. Yet I'm here to tell you that food addiction can be broken. I've discovered that there are two "escape routes" located at different stages of the cycle. One of them I have taken many times myself. The other I have uncovered through much research and prayer, and I offer it as a source of hope and healing.

In order to effectively access these escape routes, you must first make a thorough accounting of the emotional pain-chains you're now bound by. Chapter 5 will enable you to do that by exploring and identifying the negative emotions that are driving you to binge. With that knowledge in hand (and written down in your notebook), in chapter 6 you'll be guided along two escape routes—healthy, nondestructive ways to purge your pain. Just as life cycles that are broken end in death, death cycles that are broken can restore life! Jesus said in the Bible, "I have come that they might have life and have it abundantly." Hold on tight to that offer!

Lana's Story of Hope

Hi, my name is Lana, and I'm…a food addict. Wow, it's hard to put that into writing, even after knowing the truth of my addiction for more than a year now. I think it would help you to understand my journey if I go back to the beginning.

I've had a dysfunctional, love–hate affair with food ever since I can remember. I was adopted at three months old and was very tiny as a child, so my parents were always trying to get me to eat. Ours was a strict household, and my parents, I'm sure with the best intentions, would not take "no more" for an answer. Often I would sit at the table for hours after meals because I hadn't finished my plate. I can even remember a time when I had to eat a reheated dinner for breakfast because I hadn't finished it the night before.

It was about first grade that my aversion to food became an obsession with food. I would come home from school looking for my favorite foods and closet myself in my room with a snack and a book. That cycle continued well into adulthood. I had loving parents, but I often struggled with feeling "different" because of being adopted. Though I always felt that God's love and forgiveness was for the whole world, I had a hard time believing it was for me personally. This fed into my need for love and approval, and when I didn't feel that love, I'd eat to numb the pain.

In high school I would go from bingeing to fasting, and this unhealthy cycle kept my weight at a reasonably normal level (around 20 pounds overweight) until my first year in college. At that point, I had a painful experience that sent me into an emotional tailspin. I was attending a Christian college, and a person in authority sexually harassed me. I had been raised in such a strict home that I was afraid to tell anyone or ask for help because I thought I would be blamed. I lived in fear for many months until an outside speaker came to our college to speak in chapel, and something in her eyes told me I could trust her. I asked for her help, and she walked me through the journey of getting help and getting free of the harassment.

This was a crisis point for me. All of a sudden, I lost the ability to stop eating. I wasn't even able to use my unhealthy pattern of fasting anymore. I ate in secret, I ate in public, I drove out in the middle of the night to get my favorite foods—I just couldn't stop. Within two years, I gained 50 pounds.

⚜

At this point, I married my wonderful husband. I really believed that would solve my problems. I thought the loneliness I felt would no longer be a problem. How wrong I was! I didn't know that the loneliness was not from the lack of wonderful people in my life—it was coming from a broken place inside me, a place only Jesus could touch. While I had received Jesus' forgiveness and salvation as a young girl, I often felt far away from Him, fearing I wasn't good enough to be truly close to Him. I was always looking for the next and better spiritual "miracle," hoping that would touch the deep ache inside me. Although nothing made a sudden change, all the things God brought into my life began to make slow changes in me, bringing me closer and closer to the moment when He would open my eyes.

About four years ago, God began working inside me to help me face my issues with food. I had tried many diets over the years, but none had worked. In fact, I had never actually lost weight on any diet. While others lost weight, I just gained.

I began to ask for His help and open my heart to any solution that would save me from this life lived solely for the god of food. Within a month or so, the cable TV channel A&E launched a new show called *Intervention*, a show where the cameras follow someone who is an addict, show how it's destroying their life, and then record their families having an intervention with them to try to get them into treatment. I'll never forget the Sunday night I watched that show for the first time. I was in bed watching TV next to my sleeping husband, eating my usual late-night snack. The episode was about a woman with three children who was an alcoholic. It showed her pouring straight vodka into her travel mug in the morning and driving her kids to school, drinking while she drove.

By the time the show was over and the woman had agreed to go to treatment, I was sobbing so hard, I was afraid I'd wake my husband. I went into the living room, got down on my knees, and asked God, "Why am I so upset?" The answer came right away—I knew I was addicted to food, and I desperately wished someone would do an intervention with me. By this time, I weighed 300 pounds and knew my addiction would kill me...as surely as the addiction to alcohol could kill the woman I'd watched on TV. I needed help.

It felt so good to finally admit I couldn't do this myself. I knew deep down in my heart I couldn't overcome this—no diet I knew would save me, because my desire to eat was too great. This is what prompted me to look for a rehab program for people addicted to food. After three weeks of surfing the net and probably 50 phone calls to rehab centers, I found a place nearby that could take me. The price was so high that I knew I needed to make sure my insurance would pay—but when I called, they told me insurance only covered you if you were purging. I actually cried during that phone call. I felt totally alone.

Then a friend reminded me that some hospitals run a medically supervised "fast" where you eat only their food—nutrition bars, drinks, and soups. It seemed like my last resort, so I was willing to drive an hour and 15 minutes each way once a week to try to make this work. Over nine months, I lost 50 pounds on this plan, which was a great step for me as I had never lost weight on a diet before. I can vividly remember talking to my doctor the day before I started eating regular food again and saying, "I'm so scared. I'm afraid once I start eating regular food again, I won't stop." She brushed that off, but I was right. Once I started eating regular food, my addiction kicked in again, and I was off to the races. I had no idea why I couldn't stop eating, because I didn't understand I was an addict. Within a year, I had gained all that weight back plus 22 pounds more, bringing me to my all-time high of 322 pounds.

Not only was I back to the physical limitations and struggles I'd experienced before my weight loss, the self-loathing I felt was paralyzing. I had put all my effort and heart into this, and now I was failing again. Then in June 2007 I was walking really fast into a darkened movie theater, and I fell. What would have been a small amount of bruising and a minor inconvenience for a person of normal weight turned into a life-threatening injury for me. My leg swelled up and turned black from my toes to my hip. The pain from the swelling was so overwhelming that I had to go on pain medication. I very nearly had to have surgery to relieve the swelling, since my overloaded lymph system was not able to carry all the fluid from the swelling away from the injury site. It was three weeks in bed, followed by three more weeks on crutches, and almost four months before I was able to get around again without pain.

It was after this injury that I began to ask God for a solution in earnest. It hit home yet again that this addiction would kill me if I didn't get help. I began spending regular time talking with God, something I had always struggled to do in the past. I shared openly with my close friends and church family that I needed help. Finally in November 2007, God reached out and touched me deep inside my soul. While reading my Bible and worshiping I felt His presence closer to me than ever before. I felt His unconditional love more deeply than I imagined possible, and without any self-hatred I admitted to myself that my addiction to food was wasting my life, and I begged Him to help me give up my own will and trust Him to lead me out of the dark place where I was living.

Three days later, a close friend who had been in recovery from alcoholism for 12 years told me, "You're an addict, and you need to go to a recovery program. Did you know there's a group for food addicts that's based on the same principles as AA? It's called Overeaters Anonymous." That day, I found a local meeting and began to attend. I spent the first three meetings crying. Gradually I realized I had finally found a group of people who understood the battle of a true addict, and they offered me a safe place where I could begin the process of becoming rigorously honest toward myself and others. I got a sponsor (a mentor) and began working through the 12 Steps to Recovery, which helped me begin to change my life. And of course my eating habits changed as well.

Working through the first step in the 12 Steps was the most difficult: "We admitted we were powerless over food and our lives had become unmanageable." This was a challenge for me. I always thought that as a Christian I couldn't allow myself to be powerless over anything. What I didn't realize was that Christ had power, but in and of myself, I had no ability to stop eating. Once I realized that the 12 Steps were actually based in the principles of the Bible, I began to see God's truth written all over my recovery. I began to accept that, like an alcoholic, I would always have this challenge with food—my submission to God's truth has allowed me to accept that there are certain things that can never pass my lips again, else I will relapse back into my addiction. With the help of my friends who are on the same recovery road, and with God's power, I lost 56 pounds during 2008.

In the last four months, I have struggled. I've gained a little of that weight back, and the fear I felt at this setback almost made me give up. Every week at my Overeaters Anonymous meeting I would have a crisis where I'd have to decide if I would be absolutely honest or not. By the grace of God, I have been honest at every single meeting. I've continued to attend meetings and get together with others who are in recovery. I'm still working through the Steps and have now begun to regain my abstinence. What's the difference this time? I've made a choice. I've accepted that I'm not one of those who can just go on a diet and wave my weight problem goodbye. I'm an addict who needs recovery for *life*. I will not give up—because the love of Christ doesn't give up on me.

Essential in my continued recovery is taking care of myself on many levels. Regular visits to the doctor are important to this process, and a recent visit revealed that a medication I began taking four months ago has been increasing my appetite. What a gift to find out that a change in medication can help with my recovery! If I had given in to despair and stopped working toward my recovery or taking care of myself, I never would have realized how important medical care can be in my ability to live a life free of addiction.

I cannot do this alone. The shame of my addiction kept me isolated for so long. I know the path to long-term healing can only be traveled in the company of others. In Overeaters Anonymous, there is no set eating plan, only "three meals a day, nothing in between, one day at a time," unless a health issue requires snacks. The challenge of this very flexible plan is that I *cannot* follow it with my will alone. My desire to eat will always lead me to eat foods that might send me back to addiction, so I'll always need to work with a sponsor and take advantage of the help of others who are in recovery.

There are times when well-meaning Christians criticize my decision to become involved in Overeaters Anonymous. They believe a Christian can be completely free from an addiction and should never accept the identity of an addict. I respect their view, but I believe that like the apostle Paul, "If I must boast, I will boast of the things that show my weakness" (2 Corinthians 11:30). Why? Because it is a much bigger proof of God's power to show people that my life has changed inside and out...than that I could just stick to a diet long enough to get into a bathing suit.

I don't know everything about recovering from a food addiction. I think I'm just beginning that journey. What I know for certain is that humbling myself and admitting that I'm powerless over my addiction has opened up the storehouse of heaven's love in my heart. I experience the acceptance of God and the presence of Jesus on a regular basis. I'm learning to quiet my mind and heart and experience God in silence and peace. I love this new life, and by God's grace, I won't go back to the old one. This is a decision I make...one day at a time.

Chapter 5

Stuffing Down Your Emotions with Food

Food will never fix your problems.

In the last chapter we established the fact that food addictions are fueled by emotional pain—or a hungry heart, as I prefer to call it. Your heart and mind inherently sense emptiness, and they create within you an overwhelming drive to fill that emptiness with something. You've chosen food.

Daily living can cause significant emotional turmoil for an emotionally hungry person. Because raw emotions lie unhealed, just beneath your "emotional surface," they are easily inflamed by situations that would likely not affect a full-hearted, emotionally sound person to the same degree. As a result of this raw pain, you self-medicate with food—anything to make that emotion stop. Abusing food stuffs down those disturbing feelings, way down, so they stay out of sight and hopefully out of mind.

Many of us who have endured difficult emotional times would rather not think about them. *That was in the past,* you tell yourself. *I can move beyond that stuff.* So you pick yourself up by your bootstraps and march forward into the future, never casting a single glance backward. (I'm deliberately using an awkward word picture.) If you were to pause for a moment and look back over your shoulder, however, you would see it wasn't just your bootstraps you'd carried into your future! You're dragging a heavy suitcase behind you loaded with pain, raw and undealt with. By choosing not to consider that you still have "junk in your trunk," you're simply denying its powerful influence over you.

And denial is never a good thing. (See chapter 6 for more on denial.) Breaking free from compulsive overeating will only occur after you've cut yourself loose from what you're now dragging behind you.

Problem is, ignoring your pain won't make its hold on you disappear any more than ignoring a whining child will make *him* disappear. I am a big fan of Beth Moore's Bible studies. Recently I came across a quote that speaks directly to the "Why should I face my past?" question. Beth declares,

> We must be honest about where we *are* before we can journey effectively to where we want to be.[1]

Now, you and I both know where you want to be: free from the drive to overeat. Yet in order to get there, you must analyze each emotional "chain" that holds you in bondage to food so you can learn how to unlock them and get yourself free!

☙❦❧

Throughout this chapter we'll be seeking to uncover possible causes for the emotional hunger that manifests itself in your overeating behavior—"holes in your heart," if you will. This is no blame game or witch hunt. Rather, you're about to search your life for hurts that were never healed—those cavernous "heart wounds." We're also looking for any seemingly healed-over emotional wounds that, while "closed" on the surface, are in fact infected abscesses below. (Graphic, I know. But just as deadly as a festering injury.)

Looking at it another way, the emotional hurts of your past— even those in your immediate present—are like bunches of garbage in a compost heap. If they are piled up and left untended, they will rot in such a way as to stink to high heaven and will never be useful for fertilizer. In order to end up with something useful, garbage in a compost heap must be turned over, again and again. Only then can a healthy form of breakdown occur. This process of turning over and over converts your useless garbage into beneficial compost, capable of nourishment. As you process your own emotional garbage—which has left you with the "stinky" outcome of food addiction—I'll show you how you can turn your emotional trash into life treasure. Also, I'll point you to ways to fill your empty heart—but not with food this time. There's something much more satisfying for you!

At this point, please pick up your notebook—the same one you used in chapter 2. Come along with me on a trip down the aisles of "Pain-Mart." (Not a fun excursion, but fully necessary.) Browse through the selections of potential heart-hurts we'll pass by below. When you see something you identify with, place it into your cart—your notebook—so you can work on it in the next chapter. (The "Journal Time" reminder box at the end of each section are prompts to remind you to write things down.) Once you've compiled a list, short or long, we'll go through some processes of mind and soul rehabilitation in chapters 6 and 7—clinically effective processes—intended to bring complete healing to your emotional wounds.

Once Abused, Always Abused?

Do you have vivid memories of childhood abuse? Did one or both of your parents rule the home with a heavy hand? Did you live in fear of their rage, and hide in your room or flee your home to avoid their wrath? Was their punishment of you excessive, cruel, or unusual? Did you have to tiptoe around a volatile alcoholic parent? Have you endured years of verbal abuse from your caregivers, such as name calling, chastisement, and ridicule? Or perhaps you were sexually violated by a family member, relative, friend, or stranger who then threatened you to keep silent. Maybe you are still keeping silent to this day...

If this is you today, your childhood abuse cut deep and left obvious scars on your life. The deep sense of shame and loss of self-worth you feel can be nearly suffocating. I want you to know that your wounds are not so deep that they cannot be healed. There is help, and there is hope for you. Given a sound biblical method to process your pain, you will be able to effectively purge the accompanying negative emotions and behaviors that have been eating away at your heart and your health because of past abuse. This healing process will allow you to fill your heart with good things (chapter 7) instead of your stomach with harmful amounts of food. But determine not to continue abusing yourself with food, just because someone else abused you in the past. You've endured enough harm for a lifetime. Don't allow this abusive way of life to continue any longer—and certainly not at your own hands.

JOURNAL TIME

An "Out of Order" Upbringing

Did your upbringing leave you with emotional scars? Mine sure did. First of all, my childhood home was filled with arguing, critical comments, and "cheap shots"—we all (parents and siblings alike) made fun of one another mercilessly. Laughter at another's expense was not frowned upon, it was openly encouraged. My home had a "hurt someone with your words before they hurt you" environment. If I could keep the jokes targeted on someone else, I would escape becoming the target. Understandably, my upbringing created feelings of insecurity in me. It also gave me a critical spirit and a cutting tongue.

In addition, I never remember a time when my parents actually got along (except for feigned harmony around company). This disharmony created continual tension within our home and inside my stomach. It caused me to act out in school and reflect the same disrespect toward my teachers that I saw displayed toward me by my parents in our home. Dinners at my house were served with a side dish of "agita," which is the Italian slang word for agitation or anxiety. As I entered adulthood, I needed to learn how to process these emotions (and others). If I didn't, I knew they would surely swallow me alive. Later I'll share with you the pathway I took toward emotional healing. But for now let's talk about you.

What was your childhood like? Maybe yours had side dishes of other kinds of *agita*. Were your parents overcontrolling? I've known people who were raised by what I jokingly refer to as "hover mothers."

These moms hover like helicopters above their children's lives, controlling every aspect—making sure the Play-Doh colors are never mixed, choosing who their child's best friend will be, and telling them the exact time at which they should wipe their mouths during dinner. "Army sergeant" dads are equally upsetting to live with. If you were raised "in the army," then you know what it feels like to grow up never doing anything well enough or fast enough. Overcontrolling caregivers can produce deep feelings of anger and resentment in children. Insecurity and self-doubt can also result.

In the United States today, over half of all marriages end in divorce. Many wounded children have been left behind. Are you one of them? Divorce can have devastating effects on a child. The "time heals all wounds" theory, just like evolutionary theory, is chock full of holes. In fact, studies have shown quite the opposite to be true. The further from the time of a divorce a child is, the more depressed and emotionally disturbed he or she becomes.[2] The fact is, most children from divorced homes feel abandoned (by one parent), angry, insecure, and even partially responsible.

Other possible situations that may have left you with a wounded heart are poverty, racial prejudice, neglect (as we spoke of in the last chapter), and sibling rivalry or favoritism—namely you were not the "golden child," and no amount of climbing over your sibling would change that. Each of these can leave you questioning your self-worth for the rest of your life. As is commonly known, low self-esteem is at the core of most addictions. You may even be suffering from more than one addiction simultaneously, such as overeating and workaholism, just to prove to yourself and others that you're indeed worthwhile.

JOURNAL TIME

Picking Up the Pieces of Your Broken Dreams

Some of you had a pretty decent upbringing. I've met numerous adults who describe their childhood homes as resembling the 1960s television show *Leave it to Beaver.* Only well into your adulthood did you encounter a problem with overeating or overweight. On one dreadful day, the dreams you had for your life were altered. (It tightens up your throat just thinking about it.) Something so devastating happened that it sent you spiraling out of control. And you landed smack in the middle of a food addiction.

Among such possible life-altering events are: You lost your unborn baby because of a miscarriage (or two or three), your young child died, you discovered your spouse was cheating on you, your marriage ended in divorce, your unwed daughter became pregnant, your son was killed while serving his country or, worse, as the result of a crime, your teenager is addicted to drugs or alcohol, or—every parent's nightmare—he or she committed suicide.

I have walked alongside many whose lives have been permanently altered by such sorrows. While some have sought comfort in food (or other addictions), others have successfully survived without causing further harm to themselves. That is my hope for you: healing—not harming. The God of the Bible offers you this promise:

> When you pass through the waters,
> I will be with you;
> and when you pass through the rivers,
> they will not sweep over you.
> When you walk through the fire,
> you will not be burned;
> the flames will not set you ablaze. For I am the LORD, your God,
> the Holy One of Israel, your Savior.

> —ISAIAH 43:2-3

Perhaps it's not what happened to you that caused your dreams to break. Maybe it's what *hasn't* happened. Have you been waiting all your life for the perfect soul mate, and now you're nearing 40 and that person is nowhere to be found? Possibly you and your spouse envisioned a home filled with boisterous kids, but you've been unable to get pregnant or maintain your pregnancies. Maybe you do have children, but one suffers with a health problem or disability, and you've had to mourn the loss of your "perfect" child and your storybook life. Life as you had imagined it has failed to materialize.

Think carefully about this issue. It's sometimes more difficult to identify emotional pain you're carrying from something you longed to have but never did get. Write down everything that comes to mind in this category. If nothing comes at first, give yourself five or ten extra minutes to think on it. Give yourself time to scan through all your life's expectations—even the ones that seem "less tragic" in the grand scheme. Here's one possibility: What about not being able to stay home and raise your children because your income is desperately needed? Don't discount "smaller" life disappointments such as this. It could be one of the reasons you are driven to overeat.

JOURNAL TIME

Enduring Difficult Relationships

In my life the worst pain to process is the one that keeps reoccurring! If that person would just quit hurting my feelings, maybe I could move past the pain into healing. You likely feel the same way. Some of you may be enduring a difficult marriage partner. Others may live with unruly children who challenge every word and break every house rule. Comedian Jeff Allen, in one of his routines, says this about his son's disrespect: "The Bible says nothing about the age at which Satan rejected God's authority—but if I had to hazard a guess, I'd say he was about 15!" Many of you know exactly what Jeff is talking about. Parenting a rebellious teen is like trying to control a tornado blowing through your home!

For me, and possibly for you, my thorn in the flesh continues to be the mother–daughter relationship. If you had trouble getting along with your mom or dad, you may now find yourself trapped in the same tangled web. In my case, the difficulty lies in the brokenness of my mom, as I mentioned earlier. In order to stay clear of addiction, I've had to remind myself over and over again that *hurt people hurt people*. They simply are unable to choose another way of relating.

Don't forget to examine your workplace, church, and volunteer relationships. Some of the people you work alongside can send you swimming in stress soup! One man I knew allowed his workplace relationships to rob him, and subsequently his family, of decades of health and happiness. It was sad to see the obesity he took on trying to soothe himself with food become a fate shared with one of his children. And that child never even stepped foot in the father's workplace! Yet the two of them will continue to fight the battle of the bulge for the rest of their lives if they do not achieve emotional healing.

Another hugely stressful relationship problem many people must endure began when they moved next door to "the neighbor from (the nether regions)." These neighbors have proved to be unreasonable, arrogant, and selfish. (No, I don't know your neighbor, but I do know others like them.) If you could, you'd move (or blow up their house), but that's not a possibility. I know dreaming of bombings makes addiction worse, not better, but I do want you to be honest about the intensity of your feelings here—not keep them stuffed down under a meal of fried chicken!

Even your friends, your pals, your girlfriends—the very people you've invited into your life, can become a source of stress and strife. No relationship is without its trying times. And some of your deepest wounds may have been inflicted by someone you deeply trusted. I had an acquaintance in college whose mother was betrayed by both her best friend and her husband when they committed adultery together. The pain of betrayal happens, but either your response to it can take you down a pathway of addiction (to further pain and shame)…or it can become like a jagged ceramic shard, to be set alongside the other broken pieces of your past to create a beautiful life mosaic. The choice is yours…you can be broken, or you can become beautiful. (So how's your list coming along? Is it time to sharpen your pencil?)

JOURNAL TIME

Out of the Depths of Depression

Oh, man—am I familiar with this one! I can't recall a time when my mother didn't suffer from depression to one degree or another. When I was younger, she would plunge in and out of tears and despair. A dark cloud was always over her head. However, as I told you earlier, on the day that her older sister died from cancer my mother fell into a deep depression from which she was unable to pull herself out. That was the day my mom and I exchanged roles. Since my late teenage years she has taken many psychological medications, has undergone countless hours of counseling, and has twice been admitted to the psychiatric ward of the hospital. She's threatened to commit suicide hundreds of times (to this day) though, thankfully, she has never actually attempted it.

As difficult as it is to live with a depressed person, I well realize it's many times more difficult to *be* the depressed person. If you suffer from depression, either cyclically or constantly to one degree or another, consider what I mentioned previously: Psychiatrists believe that *depression is the emotion of anger turned inward*. If you are depressed, you need to identify exactly what you are angry about. But identification is not enough. My mother was fully aware of everything she was angry about and everyone she was angry with—and she made that well known to her family and counselors. The reason her acknowledgment of anger-including events, situations, and people didn't bring her any freedom is because instead of following helpful, healing counsel, she seemed determined to hold onto her pain, reliving every hurtful moment.

The feeling of utter hopelessness may be painfully familiar to you. You may be sinking under the load—all the time unaware that the reason your life seems too heavy to bear is because you are dragging an overloaded, anger-filled suitcase behind you. It will be impossible for you to lose weight if depression is your constant companion because the road of a depressed person's life, more often than not, leads to the refrigerator door.

JOURNAL TIME

Cooling Off Your Anger

Outwardly displayed anger can take many forms. You may find yourself experiencing fits of rage, directed toward the person right in front of you or at the car that just cut you off! Other times outward anger takes the form of biting sarcasm or harsh criticism. Many angry people seem to seethe with frustration at just about everything and everybody. A small adverse event can lead to an oversized volcanic eruption of anger.

Then there's that undercover form of anger known as passive–aggressive behavior. Someone who has a passive–aggressive nature thinks they have their anger hidden. Yet it's obvious to most onlookers that they indeed have "issues." This can be a tricky personality disorder to describe, so I'll go right to the dictionary for this one:

> the habitual passive resistance to demands for adequate performance in occupational or social situations, as by procrastination, stubbornness, sullenness, and inefficiency.

Simply put, this angry fellow doesn't want anyone to boss him around, so he masks his anger by putting up nonconfrontational resistance as a way of making the other person feel just as frustrated as he is. Misery loves company!

Am I describing you here? Over 25 years ago I was forced to admit I was controlled by my anger. I struggled for most of my teenage and young-adult years with tremendous resentment, directed primarily at my father. It never turned inward to become depression, but boy, did it turn outward—into rage, sarcasm, and the like. No one could set me off like my dad.

It took a while, but I am now free from the chains of chronic anger—I have been for decades now. And I was loosed from the bondage before my father passed away. His behavior never changed, but mine did. (I can't wait to tell you in the next chapter how I broke free from those heavy chains!) I came to find that when emotional (and spiritual) healing does occur, further hurts encountered tend to stick less, and slide off more easily.

By the way, be specific when jotting down notes on your emotional issues. Don't just simply write "Anger." Write down all the *reasons* for your anger that come to mind. This will prove useful for when you work through each one.

JOURNAL TIME

The Stress of Success

I'm willing to bet that your day-to-day work life is filled with plenty of its own stresses. These workday pressures may well be the ones that push you over the edge, jump-starting your cycle of using food as a tranquilizer. If you are a stay-at-home mom and homemaker, while you don't have to answer to a boss or make payroll for your employees, you are in no way exempt from feeling overwhelmed by the demands on your time, frustrated by those little ones in your midst, and hopelessly behind on your to-do list. There never seems to be an end to your day (which often can continue on through the night—am I right?). If your job is done well, some days your good parenting can feel like it's going to be the death of you!

Over the past decade the trend has been for companies to cut back on their staff, which places higher demands on their remaining employees. The length of a work day for many has extended from eight hours to ten. Add to that multiple hours of commuting, and by the day's end you may be fit to be tied. Even if you are your own boss (as I am), and your commute is confined to within your own home (as mine typically is) you realize you're squeezing out every last bit of yourself so you can produce more work in a shorter period of time.

Or perhaps, like me again, you're juggling multiple job tasks within the same week. Talk about stress—some days I forget which hat I'm supposed to have on! Funny story: My daughter had a school project in which she had to select one of her parents and interview them regarding their occupation. She then had to create a poster board depicting the parent's occupation for display in her classroom. She chose me. Big mistake! After about an hour of interviewing me, she had a fourfold occupation board to design. She was not happy. Frustrated, she whined, "Why can't you be like other mothers and have just one or two jobs?" (I told her she should have interviewed her father!)

Time in the workplace has changed greatly during the last 20 years. Back when I first started working after college, I had a lunch *hour*. Now, as do many others, I break to eat for 10 minutes and then head right back to work. More in less time—that seems to be the theme of this decade. Many of us fall victim to it. When you return home from a high-paced, jam-packed day, what do you do? Do you head straight to the refrigerator? Maybe you don't even make it home without first swinging through the drive-thru window for a snack to "take the edge off." Have you ever said to yourself, *I deserve this! What a day I had!* If so, you can add workday stress to your tally of the emotions you're trying to stuff down with food.

Lastly I want to mention another area of "work" that may be adding to your daily stress level. That is volunteering. We all want to do a good job at what we've volunteered to do, and likely you volunteered because you were passionate about whatever you got yourself involved in. You may work with a Brownie troop or as a youth-group sponsor. Maybe you run a vital component of a community outreach program or, on top of everything else, have to prepare weekly to teach a Sunday-school class full of rowdy kids. Just admit to yourself, if need be, that part of your emotional stress may be coming from *any* commitment in which you feel overwhelmed. So don't feel guilty to write down your volunteer position. It doesn't mean you'll have to quit. It only means you have to learn a better method to cope.

JOURNAL TIME

Financial Woes

Money worries and overeating are common companions. I write at a time when the financial future is not looking so bright. The stock market has dropped significantly. Job-loss and unemployment rates are rising. Housing foreclosures are everywhere. Everyday people like me seem to have lost faith in those whose job it is to make these big financial decisions.

The stage is set for some serious financial worries—the kind that drive you to eat if you're not careful. Will you have a job? Can you pay your bills? What will happen to your retirement savings? And on and on. If you feel yourself suddenly getting hungry every time you compare your bills to your bank statements or each time you open your investment statements (or wishing you had enough money to have investments), then place financial stress on your list as an emotion you are trying to stuff down along with that sandwich. The ironic thing about overeating when you're worried about money is that it costs you more money! But then again, whoever said food addiction was a reasonable behavior? Good news for your bottom line—help begins in the next chapter. Press on, we're almost there.

JOURNAL TIME

The Plague of Fear

It seems like fear and anxiety plague more and more people. Some of you may have very realistic fears, such as wondering about the disabling effects of a disease you've been diagnosed with, questioning when you'll find another job after being laid off, or fretting over the crumbling life of your child who you recently discovered is into drugs or pornography.

You are completely within your rights to feel the way you do. This exercise isn't about judging the validity of your emotions. It's about uncovering and naming any potentially harmful emotion, many of which you have come by honestly. You need to be able to experience these negative emotions and work though them without having to turn to an addictive agent to help you manage. That's where this book comes into play.

Some fears are rational; others are not. Some people are worry-warts, plain and simple. They make up things to worry about. They turn molehills into mountains. For example, do you question the faithfulness of your spouse when you have no good reason to do so? Are you in constant dread each day you go into work, wondering if it will be your last even though there hasn't been any talk of layoffs? Do you fear going to the doctor because you may be diagnosed with a dread disease? Do you need to admit that you've made up highly detailed, full-blown scenarios of devastating events in your own mind and then rehearsed them over and over again, day and night (including your reaction to them)?

There's no doubt that this sort of behavior is unhealthy for your waistline. In chapter 8 I will tackle the issue of conquering a negative thought life with a thoroughly proven method—one I've had to use on myself over and over again (still to this day). Regardless of the source, fear and anxiety, real or imagined, can surely cause you to pack on the pounds if you fail to find another way of comforting yourself. My hope is that you'll discover there's a much better way.

JOURNAL TIME

Thinking Less of Yourself

Are you willing to admit that you feel insecure and maybe even undeserving of anyone's love and attention from time to time—or, sadly, all of the time? Do you feel inadequate in this world, failing to measure up to those around you? Maybe the people in your life who you looked up to have convinced you that you have little value—and over time you've allowed yourself to agree with them.

If you've been brought to see yourself as less than who you were created to be, then shame on those who stole your self-worth! According to the Bible, you were created in God's image, for His enjoyment. Jesus went to the cross with your name written on His heart, taking your place, taking the punishment for your sins. He longs to have a close friendship with *you*. Scripture says God knows the very number of hairs on your head (both before and after you brush them.) His gaze is always upon you. He is absolutely, 100 percent in love with you. So please don't overeat under the guise of "I don't deserve to be healthy... happy...loved." If you do, you've fallen for a lie. You deserve much more. In fact, you deserve everything God intended to give you.

JOURNAL TIME

As your notebook likely testifies, food addiction can have many emotional roots. In the next few chapters we will begin plowing a new garden for your life, one which will be prepared to grow healthy thoughts, actions, and reactions. So gather your pick and hoe—there's much hardened ground to be turned over (old ways), many weeds and roots to remove (negative thoughts and emotional hurts), and many stones to be discarded (your addiction) before we can plant new, tender shoots (the new you!). The Bible says a man reaps what he sows. Let's begin to sow health so you can reap life in full abundance!

A Midbook Assignment for You

Now that you've had a chance to delve into what might really be at the heart of your emotional eating, I'd like you to begin a weeklong project. Authors of diet books and diet plans often ask you to maintain a food journal so you can keep track of everything you eat and drink throughout your day.

I'd like you to think about keeping a different type of "food journal." It's actually not a food journal, but rather an emotions journal as it relates to your eating. Record your felt emotions both before and after you eat, whether a full meal, a snack you grab on the go, or even a milkshake you down in the car on your long commute home. Do write down what you ate, but more important, record how you felt before you grabbed some-thing to eat and then how you felt emotionally afterward. "Keeping an 'emotional eating journal' sounds kind of weird, Lisa. I never think before I eat—I just eat!" This process does sound out of the ordinary, but isn't that what you're looking for, a new approach to your long-term problem? Simply keep a running list of how you feel and what you're driven to eat (and how much) as a result. Don't forget to note the aftereffect on your emotions. Here's a suggested question: Do you feel calmer and more at ease, or do you feel guilty or ashamed? You can develop your own.

What you need to understand is exactly how your negative emotions are playing into your overeating behavior. The best way to come face-to-face with this premise is to see it for yourself. A friend of mine, when asked to do this exercise, realized after only three days that every time she felt angry, she headed to the freezer for a bowl of ice cream. Eating ice cream was her coping mechanism for dealing with her out-of-control emotion of anger. Unfortunately, along with obesity, that behavior increased her blood pressure and blood-sugar levels as well. Not the best way to cope, was it?

It's so common for people to try to stuff down unpleasant emotions every time they arise with the pleasure of food or drink, and never make the connection between their emotions and their overeating. You have the chance to deal with your emotions in a way that leaves you healthier, not sicker.

You can start today. In your journal notebook, make a chart like the one shown below. For the next week, fill it in every time you put something (other than water) in your mouth. Don't fret if you forget one day—simply continue until you have seven days of data recorded. Be careful to record not the situation, but rather the way the situation made you feel.

For example, if your teenager screamed at you for forgetting to pick her up after school, and you argued angrily over it, you could get away with writing down "angry" as your emotion before downing the jelly donut. However, a more accurate assessment of the underlying reason for your anger might be the feeling of inadequacy as a mother that your teenager made you experience. You may even want to tune into your self-talk at this point. It may sound something like this: *I'm so pathetic that I can't even remember to pick up my kid after school. I'll never be able to satisfy my child's needs.*

Day 1	Emotion before eating	Foods/ approximate quantity eaten	Emotion after eating

After keeping track of your emotions for a week, you'll begin to notice some patterns emerge. One thing you'll see for sure (as did my friend) is just how much you rely on food to lift you out of your emotional pit.

Now let's move onto the next chapter and figure out how to process the harmful emotions of your past (journaled throughout chapter 5) and how to cope with the emotions of your present (from your emotional eating chart above).

Chapter 6

Healthy Ways to Purge Your Pain

Resolving your hurts will release your healing.

There is tremendous freedom waiting for you if you diligently process and purge the negative emotional situations and feelings you documented in your journal while reading the last chapter. The word *purge* is often used in a negative sense today, and is typically associated with the act of vomiting or abuse of laxatives after a person binges on food. However, a more balanced definition is "to get rid of, to remove or purify by way of a cleansing process." It's this cleansing form of purging that I'd like to spend time on in this chapter. No more stuffing down, pushing aside, or hiding away your pain—it's finally time to off-load the heavy weight you've been carrying around—the emotional weight first, followed by the physical.

In chapter 4, where we explored the food-addiction cycle, I mentioned two "escape routes" that lie hidden within this cycle. Before we start in with them, I'd like to address those of you who are still unsure whether "food addict" actually applies to you. It still sounds harsh and very...*extreme*. Even though you're overweight or obese, you don't actually have an *addiction* problem, you believe—you could stop your destructive behavior of overeating whenever you want. You simply haven't chosen to do so yet.

Do you tell yourself that you just happen to love food—its aroma and texture, and the way it tastes—and you're merely enjoying all the good things to eat that God has placed here on this earth? Have you found yourself explaining to others that your metabolism has always been slow? You were born chunky and you still haven't lost all your baby fat...Everyone in your family is "big-boned"...You don't even know why you are overweight—you eat so very little. Have you ever said any of these (aloud or to yourself)?

Don't answer this next question right away—just chew on it awhile. Could it be possible you're denying your food-addiction problem or the effect of your past or present on your eating, because you're fearful— fearful that if you let your guard down and "go there," you'll be unable to resolve anything? So rather than be faced with uncertainty, help- lessness, or outright failure to resolve your emotional pain or addictive behavior, it just works better to deny (whether consciously or subcon- sciously) that this problem is yours.

A psychotherapist friend of mine, Scott Forsmith, made a crucial comment when I was interviewing him for this book. Please listen to it. He said, "You can only *heal* what you allow yourself to *feel*." Stop and read it again. If you're struggling with being overweight, if you have yo-yoed up and down or have been on numerous diets without long-term change...consider dropping your guard and allowing your- self to *feel* what it is you need to *heal* from. I urge you to give special attention to this chapter. You can benefit greatly from some processing help. And you'll find it right here. So please don't skip over anything or turn a deaf ear.

Stepping Out in Faith: My Personal Story

To be honest with you, if it were not for my personal relationship with the Lord Jesus Christ, and if I had not studied and applied the teachings of the Holy Bible to my life, I would be one messed-up woman! People who know about the dysfunctional home I grew up in (and now you're one of them) and the trying circumstances surrounding my family have often remarked how amazed they are at "how well I turned out." Well, so am I. My response is always the same: "It's by the grace of God that I am who I am today." When I think more carefully about it, it has just as much to do with God's mercy as with His grace.

Mercy, by definition, means having something bad withheld from you that you actually did deserve to suffer. There was enough going on in my life before I decided to follow Jesus to deserve nothing but reprimand from God. By the time my teenage years rolled around, I was prideful, self-seeking, and disrespectful of my parents and teachers. I was a gossip, sported quite a foul mouth, and became sexually promiscuous at a young age. I knew what God's Word said about the life I had chosen, yet I was determined to live a life of immediate pleasure, one without rules of engagement—even if it was filled with what I knew deep inside to be sin.

When I finally came to the place where my irreverence for God and His Word broke my heart, I asked Him to forgive my sinful behaviors. And I dedicated my future to living as He had created me to live—by His ways. Friend, God showed His mercy to me (and to you) by sending His Son, Jesus, to die on the cross in order to take the penalty for our sins upon Himself. By confessing my sinfulness and by accepting His gift of eternal salvation, I gained the freedom I needed to not live a life marked by my own sinful behavior, or forever stained by the sinful and dysfunctional acts of others. God's mercy made it possible for me to not have to pay the penalty for my sins. ("The wages of sin is death"—Romans 6:23a.) That penalty, which I rightly deserved, has instead been paid in full by my Savior ("... but the gift of God is eternal life in Christ Jesus"—Romans 6:23b).

I am also the person I am today because of God's grace. *Grace* means receiving something good we don't deserve to have, such as the ability to have a personal relationship with the Creator of the universe. Such as access to His supernatural power for healing from the past and living daily lives that reflect His character. Surrendering my life to Christ has brought me true freedom and reward that I'm personally convinced is not possible any other way. ("He brought me out into a spacious place [blessed me]; he rescued me [forgave my sins and restored my life] because he delighted in me"—Psalm 18:19.)

Today I live a life full of good things from God, the greatest of which is peace—peace with God, and with my husband, children, and friends—and even peace with my past. I also have confidence that God will remain true to His promises. When hard times come—and believe me they do keep coming—I rely on the scripture verse that assures me that "We know that in all things God works for the good of *those who love him, who have been called according to his purpose*"(Romans 8:28).

I emphasized the final phrases of that verse on purpose. You see, the first part of that promise depends on the last part being true. Only after I committed myself to follow Jesus did that promise become mine! The only part of this entire process of life change that is "me" was my willingness to accept God's offer of forgiveness and my continuing desire to obey the teachings of Jesus—which I am only capable of doing under the powerful influence of God the Holy Spirit. The rest is a gift from Jesus Christ. Well, friend, that's my story, and I'm sticking with it.*

The First Escape Route

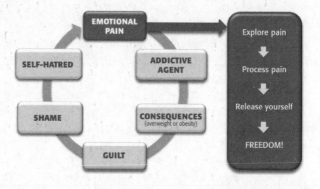

Now on to healthy ways to purge the emotional pain that's the driving force behind your food and weight troubles. The first plan of escape is available early in the addiction cycle. In fact, it has the power to keep you away from all sorts of addictions! This escape route lies between the occurrence of emotional pain (stage 1, if you will) and the choice to use an addictive agent to cover it up (stage 2).

The route is a three-part method I learned to use and have been continuing to use for decades now—as I have needed to process a *lot* of emotional turmoil. I've discovered that by carefully following this escape route, my emotional pain can be rerouted and handled in such a way that the outcome is peace and freedom rather than angst and bondage. In my experience, repeated practice of this method certainly improves my response time! This escape route will free you to spend less time lingering in your emotional pain and more time living your life to its fullest!

---

*   See "Making My Story Yours" on page 179 for a guide as to how you can take the same path I did.

Explore Your Pain

In the last chapter you noted down the significant negative life situations you've endured. Now get your journal, go back through the list you made, and attach an emotion or two that describes how you *feel* about each issue. If you find yourself using the same word over and over to describe your feelings, look through the following list and see if there isn't a better-suited "emotional tag" you can hang on each one.

Negative Feelings That Can Result from Emotional Pain	
anxious	ruined
ashamed	sad
depressed	scared
disgraced	smothered
hopeless	unlovable
hurt	unwanted
incompetent	unworthy
rejected	worried

Remember Scott Forsmith's pointed observation—"We cannot heal from anything that we will not first allow ourselves to feel"? It's not enough to just mentally *acknowledge* painful situations, past or present, as you did in the last chapter. You must bring yourself to identify with the *feelings* the situation produced in you at that time or continue to produce in you now.

Once you have successfully *named* a feeling, you must be willing to *claim* that feeling. By this I mean that you must actually give yourself the time and space to experience the identified feeling or feelings firsthand. If you noted you felt ashamed, *feel* that shame. If you were frightened, *feel* the fear. This is not acting class—this is honestly allowing yourself to get real, so you can become healed.

JOURNAL TIME

The next step after getting real with your pain is to allow yourself to *grieve* each event or situation. There are seven documented stages of grieving.[1] I'll list them below.

The Seven Stages of Grief	
Stage 1:	Shock or denial
Stage 2:	Anger
Stage 3:	Bargaining
Stage 4:	True grief
Stage 5:	Acceptance
Stage 6:	Forgiveness
Stage 7:	Resolution

This grief-processing list takes its origin from the five-stage grief cycle originally put forth by Swiss-born psychiatrist Elisabeth Kübler-Ross in her 1969 book *On Death and Dying.* I'd like to highlight a few details.

First, all grief begins with either shock or denial. You may have been shocked, surprised, or caught off guard by the hardship you endured. Or possibly you deny (or have denied in the past) that what occurred was truly a big issue. This first stage, while it can be very brief, can also endure over years and decades.

Secondly, *anger* is part of the grieving process. It is completely acceptable to get angry about your past or present circumstances. They've caused you great pain—still do. The thing about anger is that it is a *secondary emotion*. Psychotherapist Scott Forsmith explained to me that anger is the *result* of past pain, present frustration, or future fear. It's not a primary feeling. (If you look back, you'll see I didn't include it on the list of possible feelings.) If you documented that your painful events have made you "angry," you'll have to dig down a bit deeper. Some other emotion lies beneath that anger. Anger, according to Scott, is like smoke…you have to follow it back to the fire.

The final thing I want you to note is that *true* grieving only comes after the bargaining process is over. The bargaining stage is a bit curious. It can take many forms. Maybe with you, you've been hoping that if you play the rest of your life "by the book," you can overcome your past. Maybe, you reason, if you raise your own kids well, then you'll escape the negative results of your own broken life. Whatever form it takes, realize that it's in no way useful in resolving grief. It's just something you must move past.

Stages 5, 6, and 7 are what I want to home in on for the remainder of this chapter. Are you still with me?

Process Your Pain

Because people have been created with unique God-given personalities, it's not unusual that each of us may find certain ways to process our emotions to be more effective, even more appealing, than others. I won't go into depth, but I do want to highlight two well-recognized contrasting traits. If you can recognize which of the two best describes you, it will be useful in determining which way is best for you to process your emotions.

I'm referring to *extrovert* and *introvert*. Both words contain the same root, *vert*, which in Latin means "to turn." It is the prefixes that set these personality traits apart. The prefix *extra-* means "beyond." The extroverted person "turns beyond themselves," or to put it another way, they "face out into the world around them." These people love to talk to others and readily offer their stories, opinions, and ideas. If you are an extrovert, then, according to psychologists Minirth and Meier, the key to processing your emotional refuse pile will be for you to *talk through your past.*[2] You can certainly use a layperson as your sounding board, but I do suggest a trained counselor, psychologist, or psychiatrist for the best results. These people are not only equipped to listen without becoming burdened themselves, but they are also better able to direct you as you work through each tender issue. Furthermore, they are skilled in helping you avoid getting stuck in any one emotion while processing it.

If you prefer quiet, intimate social settings, or if your palms sweat when you are forced to interact with strangers, then you're likely to be what psychologists call an *introvert*, or someone who is "turned within." If that is the case then Minirth and Meier suggest you may be better off *writing your past out*, rather than talking it out. You will find you can effectively work through your emotions with lots of paper and ink. No other person may be needed! Simply start writing about each emotional topic until there's nothing left to write.

This is not a hard and fast rule—I know creative extroverts who are much better at processing the thoughts of their heart on paper than with spoken words. Also, in addition to writing it out and talking it out, many people need, on their journey toward emotional freedom, to be able to *cry it out* as well. Diane Ayars, the wife of my church's senior pastor, made a sweet analogy many years back during a talk she gave at our women's retreat. Acknowledging the need for those who are hurt to "cry it out," she gently said, "Tears are liquid words."

That was a beautiful word picture of the visceral need some of us have to simply "have a good cry." Sometimes our pain is too deep, and there are no words we can find that even begin to describe what we feel. That is when the floodgates open and the tears stream down our cheeks. I'll freely admit—been there, done that. It's all part of the healing process. If you haven't allowed yourself the freedom to weep over your emotional pain, please do. It may be the only way for you to move forward in your fight against overeating.

Some people have so much pent-up anger that they may need to *pound it out* before they can begin to chase the "smoke" back to its true source. (Some broken people physically abuse others because of a "need" they say they have to release their pain in a physical way. This is *not* what I'm speaking of.)

In the 2008 movie *Fireproof*, a frustrated husband periodically can be seen smashing away at household items using his trusty baseball bat—a garbage can, an old computer…And each time he is witnessed by his curious and somewhat shocked neighbor. Anyway, if you believe *you* would be able to move forward in your healing process better if you could "just hit something," here are a few options: 1) Find a punching bag, don a pair of boxing gloves, and begin swinging; 2) take a walk into the woods, find a big stick and an even larger tree trunk, and whack away; 3) join a kick-boxing class; or 4) grab your own bat and have at it—you against a rugged plastic garbage can (just don't let anyone see you...you may scare your neighbors!).

Letting It Out

You may have seen episodes of *The Bob Newhart Show* that depicted two people, usually a husband and wife, in a counseling session. The counselor (Newhart) would hand both of them big red sponge-bats, and the two frustrated partners would begin to wallop one another (and the surrounding furniture) with all the angst they had been keeping bottled up inside.

Here in New York where I live, I heard of a place that lets you hit baseballs into old glass window panes "just for fun." This could merely be a New Yorker's way of recreating. But why do I get the sense that more than a few of these window-smashers are saddled with their own set of anger issues? I don't know for sure—just a guess.

Release Yourself

In motivational books and lectures a story often surfaces about the method used for circus elephant training. It seems that all you need in order to train an elephant to walk in tight circles is a piece of rope and a stake. This training must begin when the elephant is young and "impressionable." The circus trainer begins by hammering a firm stake into the center of the circle around which he wants the elephant to walk. He then ties the elephant to the stake with a short length of sturdy rope. Day after day he prods the elephant to get him moving. At first the elephant tries to head off in a different direction, pulling with all his might. But alas, the rope keeps him well-tethered to the stake. So round and round he goes, day after day, month after month, year after year...

Surprisingly, after the elephant has reached full, massive maturity, because of his well-ingrained, tried-and-failed escape history, the rope can be removed. But the elephant, seeing the stake, will continue to circle it when "stimulated" to begin the daily exercise. He never tries to walk another path, because past history has "proved" it is impossible. All the while the strong, giant elephant is free to move about the circus floor, any which way he chooses, but he remains fixed to his small circular course.

Many of you will work strenuously at regaining your freedom. You'll cut the emotional cords that have held you to the stake of food addiction, but your past will fool you into believing that you cannot turn away and walk in your new direction—living life the way you always dreamed. Here's the word picture lesson I want to leave with you: Don't live like that elephant. Break your food addiction cycle and move on! Just because the refrigerator remains in your kitchen, there is no need to "circle around it" any longer. You can control food now; it no longer has to control you!

The graphic on page 106 summarizes this first escape route. Return to it as many times as you need to. There is no shame in repeating this exercise—only good sense.

The Second Escape Route

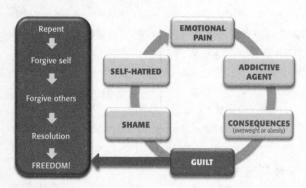

This second getaway lies at a critical juncture in the food-addiction cycle. It needs to be accessed after you feel the guilt of overeating, but before you allow yourself to move from guilt into the downward spiral of shame. Guilt is a potent emotion. It motivates its subject to react. It has the power to hold you captive in dark despair; conversely, it has the wonderful potential to lead you toward help, hope, and healing. (See the sidebar below.) The choice is yours.

The Dark and Light Side of Guilt

Guilt is a powerful emotion. When we do something we acknowledge as wrong, the normal response is for us to feel guilty. We each have been created with an internal moral compass that helps us determine when this emotion should arise (if we haven't deadened our sensitivity to it). After the onset of guilt, I believe there are two warring forces that wish to use that guilt in polar-opposite ways. On the light side, God wants to use the emotion of guilt to draw us to repentance. He wants us to acknowledge our wrongdoing, take responsibility for it, and ask Him for *His* power not to repeat it. If we handle guilt in this way, we restore our relationship to our Creator and can exist in peace and harmony with Him.

Satan and his forces (the spiritually dark side) also want to make use of the guilt you and I feel after we've done wrong. He wants to usher us right into the "Hall of Shame," where we can brood over how lame and despicable we are. In fact, if he can get us to beat up on ourselves enough, he may even be able to move us to the next stage in the cycle...self-hatred. What a sly dog he is! I guess that's why Scripture warns us in this way:

> Be self-controlled and alert. Your enemy the devil prowls around like a roaring lion looking for someone to devour (1 Peter 5:8).

Plain and simple, Satan's way leads to further bondage; God's way leads to complete freedom!

This process of breaking the cycle of food addiction will resemble in part some of the methodology used by the nationally recognized program Overeaters Anonymous. (See sidebar, "The Twelve Steps of Overeaters Anonymous.") One reason is that the process requires your *acknowledgment of a Higher Power*. For me, that Higher Power is God

Almighty, who calls himself "I AM" in the Bible, and His Son, Jesus Christ—who I happen to know on a personal basis. Another similarity is the utilization of what I will refer to as *repentance*. You'll find the act of repentance to be a necessary part of any addiction recovery (see Steps 5 and 7 in the sidebar on the next page). In fact, all the 12-Step programs were founded on biblical principles of acknowledging a higher power, repenting of wrongdoing, admitting personal weakness, and seeking strength from this Higher Power to break the addiction cycle and prevent future relapse.

Though a person can proceed along this escape route without "naming" their Higher Power, it has been my personal experience that this second escape route to freedom is most effective and long-lasting when a person begins with a heart of Christian faith. This is for two reasons. First, this escape route is based on the biblical teachings of Jesus Christ; and second, the power for change that God the Holy Spirit gives to a believer is undeniable when witnessed firsthand.

Can you utilize this method without being spiritual at all? Well, sort of—to a lesser degree. Again, sincere repentance and complete forgiveness of yourself and others are supercharged in a supernatural way when you believe fully and rely wholeheartedly on a Higher Power, who for me is the Lord Jesus Christ. I'll take you along this second escape route—see if you can better understand my conviction as we go over the process. If you choose to attempt this route without a spiritual underpinning, know that I certainly respect you and your efforts. Yet I would be disingenuous if I didn't offer you the most tried-and-true method I know—so I hope you'll respect my position as well.

The Twelve Steps of Overeaters Anonymous

1. We admitted we were powerless over food—that our lives had become unmanageable.

2. Came to believe that a Power greater than ourselves could restore us to sanity.

3. Made a decision to turn our will and our lives over to the care of God as we understood Him.

4. Made a searching and fearless moral inventory of ourselves.

5. Admitted to God, to ourselves and to another human being the exact nature of our wrongs.

6. Were entirely ready to have God remove all these defects of character.

7. Humbly asked Him to remove our shortcomings.

8. Made a list of all persons we had harmed and became willing to make amends to them all.

9. Made direct amends to such people wherever possible, except when to do so would injure them or others.

10. Continued to take personal inventory and when we were wrong, promptly admitted it.

11. Sought through prayer and meditation to improve our conscious contact with God as we understood Him, praying only for knowledge of His will for us and the power to carry that out.

12. Having had a spiritual awakening as the result of these Steps, we tried to carry this message to compulsive overeaters and to practice these principles in all our affairs.[3]

Repent

Right off the bat I'm using a churchy word. Actually, it origi-nated before the Christian faith was ever established. God (Yahweh) chose the nation of Israel, the descendants of Abraham's son Isaac, to become His favored people. They were to be set apart from the surrounding nations by the following of a strict code, or law, which governed many aspects of their daily lives. When they broke any part of the law, God directed them to *repent* of their law-conflicting ways. *Repent* in the Hebrew language means to "turn and proceed in the opposite direction."

Why am I suggesting you make repentance your first step? It's because you're presently in the Land of Guilt. And that guilt you are feeling is every bit a correct emotional response given what you have done—abuse food (and as a result, yourself). Looking at it from a Christian point of view, you acted against what the Bible has commanded you to do in two respects. 1) You have made food an idol by running to *it* for comfort instead of to God. 2) The apostle Paul charges believers to treat their physical bodies as holy and sacred, reminding us that our bodies are spiritual containers for the Holy Spirit.

So yes, you are right to feel guilty. The real question is, *Whatcha gonna do about it?* I suggest you come clean and repent—the sooner the better. The more quickly you do, the less chance you will have to circle around like that trained elephant and take the captive's next step into shame. It is as easy as saying something like this:

> *I'm so sorry, God, that I took the gift of nourishment You gave me and turned it into a harmful, addictive agent. I agree with You that my behavior is out of my control. I ask that You would forgive me and help me to make a better choice the next time… and the time after that…*

But what if you're not buying into this God thing just yet? In that case I suggest you identify with the feelings of remorse and regret for how poorly you've treated your body…after all it has done for you. It doesn't deserve to be abused and uncared for.

Forgive Yourself

For those of you who prayed the prayer of repentance (or something similar) from the last section (yes, somehow God knows who's sincere and who's just going through the motions…I guess that's what makes Him God): The much harder thing to achieve is the ability to forgive yourself. We are our own worst critics. But let me say this as plainly as I know how. If God has said we're forgiven, who are we to still hold a grudge against ourselves? To deny ourselves forgiveness when Jesus died on the cross, effectively saying, *Don't worry, I've got it covered. Your sin's on Me,* is to deny the power of His crucifixion and resurrection. It is quite simply disbelief in God. Author Beth Moore recently addressed this topic on one of her televised teaching sessions. She said that when we refuse to forgive ourselves even after we've asked God to forgive us, God doesn't look down on us and say, *Aren't you humble!* Rather, He says, *Aren't you faithless!* Who are you? Are you faithless or faith-full? Choose the latter!

The bottom line is, you need to let yourself off the hook. It does no good to add an emotional beating to the physical beating you've given your body. The bingeing episode you succumbed to is over. The past is in the past. Accept your incidental failure and move beyond it toward a better "next time." Don't drag the past with you into the future. Allow yourself to move forward...in a healthier direction.

Forgive Others

From the time I was a small child I knew the answer to my Sunday-school teacher's question: "Why do we forgive others?" Impulsive as I was, I usually forgot about the hand-raising part and would blurt out, "Because He (God) first forgave us!" Simple question, simple answer, simple mind...As I grew older and my understanding matured, I received more in-depth teaching on the subject. (I credit my church's senior pastor, Lester Ayars, with educating me on the many facets of biblical forgiveness.) In its fullness, it isn't quite as simple as I first understood it to be. Yet when boiled down to its essence my original "quick answer" is still basically the truth.

What I learned was that I had the wrong idea of what "I forgive you" means. When I forgive someone it *doesn't* mean that what they did to me (or didn't do) wasn't wrong, or that it didn't damage me in some way. Nor does it mean I'm somehow justifying their past behavior. And it doesn't always mean I need to reconcile with that person. It simply means that I'm letting them off my "hook" and placing them on God's "hook." Though that person *hurt* me, they *sinned* against my heavenly Father. I'm told in the Bible,

> Do not take revenge, my friends, but leave room for God's wrath, for it is written: "It is mine to avenge; I will repay," says the Lord (Romans 12:19).

What I'm saying is, I am no longer keeping a record of the wrongs done against me. I refuse to rehash, relive, or return to that emotional place anymore. Think about it. All those years you've been holding onto unforgiveness, churning it into bitterness and resentment, what has the perpetrator been doing? That's right—they've moved on with their broken life. They likely don't recall their shameful behavior often, if at all—*you* do! Forgiveness does far more to liberate you than it does to release the one who hurt you. This is very difficult to put into practice...I know. But I'm encouraged to respond this way because of the example Christ gave me as He hung on the cross and said, "Father, forgive them, for they do not know what they are doing" (Luke 23:34).

"Yeah—but you don't know what that person did to me!" you may be shouting at this book right now. You're right, I don't. But your heavenly Father does. He saw it, He wept when you did, and He's offering you a way out. Let Him be the Judge. That's His job—it was never meant to be yours.

There's one final suggestion I have on forgiving others. It can work equally well for anyone, regardless of spiritual bent. When dealing with present or past "people-perpetrators," or the memories thereof, I find it extremely helpful to remind myself of these facts: *Hurt people tend to hurt people.* Broken people want to break other people. People in emotional pain like to have company, so they sometimes try to bring you into their pain. When you know why someone is causing you pain, it is often easier to forgive them.

Resolution

Repent, forgive yourself, forgive others—and finally, *resolution*. In the book *Love Hunger*, Dr. Frank Minirth had this to say:

> Resolution is the opposite of resentment. Resentment is unresolved anger that continues to boil away inside, creating pressure until it can erupt in an abscess. Resolution is the sense of health, cleanliness and peace that comes from knowing that the issue has been put to rest. The problem has been solved, and I can go on from here with confidence.[4]

I think of resolution as looking forward instead of constantly glancing backward. Much like what Dr. Minirth said about moving forward with confidence. Life is to be enjoyed. Let your past go...just like that. And you can't wait until you *feel* like letting it go. Forgiveness and resolution are an act of your will, not your feelings.

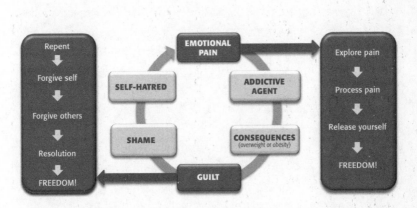

There you have it—the one-two punch to knock out your food-addiction cycle and send it spinning off! You will undoubtedly need to return to this model and remind yourself of healthy ways to purge your emotional pain rather than binge on food and jump back onto the not-so-merry-go-round. It's wonderful that you've chosen to step off this horror ride. Realize that implementing your decision to heal will take time, patience, and practice.

As you move forward in this process, the next thing you'll need to learn is how to fill your heart instead of your stomach, which is the topic of chapter 7.

Darlene's Story of Hope

My early childhood and teenage years were emotionally challenging and in some ways very damaging. My father was an alcoholic. Anger was the theme of my parents' marriage. My relationship with my mother was characterized by anger as well—she was critical of everything I did, and because I could never please her, I was yelled at much of the time.

When I was 16, my parents finally ended up divorcing (after threatening to do so since I was 12). During those four years of turbulence, a friend of mine suggested I seek counsel from a young man she knew and trusted. Tragically, the man she brought me to drugged and then raped me. I became pregnant as a result. The fear, shame, and confusion I felt left me immobilized. I was nearly six months pregnant when I finally confessed the situation to my mother. So when I was 14, my mom (acting out of her own fear and shame) immediately took me to get an abortion—believing it would be in everyone's best interest. Not so. I carried all these painful emotions with me right into my young adulthood.

When I turned 22, I moved from New York to California for what I thought would be a new beginning. Unfortunately, I couldn't escape my past or myself, and I ended up dragging my emotional pain along with me for 3000 miles! By the time I was in my mid-twenties, the comfort and escape I had been seeking from alcohol, drugs, and overeating had, instead, left me miserable and enslaved. My life had spiraled down to the point where I was struggling with depression, despair, self-hatred, and condemnation.

I hated my life, and I hated myself. I was unemployed, completely inactive, and emotionally despondent. I spent each day lying on my couch watching soap operas and planning my next meal. I grew heavier and heavier, finally reaching 200 pounds—80 pounds heavier than I should have been. The physical results of my destructive lifestyle and the shame that accompanied it lasted for several years. As I sank deeper and deeper into depression I was unable to stop my addictive cycle. I grieved over the person I had become. I was quickly losing hope, not only for myself physically, but for all of life. I was so overweight and out of control in my eating…but I knew this only reflected how out of control and defeated I felt in all the other areas of my life.

I remember the morning clearly. At 27 years old, lying on the couch, I saw myself positioned at a crossroads. Was I going to continue on this path to destruction, or would I choose another? I knew it was a matter of choosing between life and death. Buried way deep down in my heart was a "survival instinct" (which I now recognize as God's voice) that instructed me to *choose life*. I knew I wanted to live, but I also knew that what I was presently doing wasn't living. And I desperately wanted to be whole and healthy.

I had so much work to do on so many levels: emotional, physical and spiritual. So I decided that very day to work on the physical first. As horrible as it was, I tried to find a pair of sweat pants that would fit me to begin an exercise program. This alone was not an easy task, but eventually I did, and went down to a high-school track where I foolishly thought I would just start jogging. After years of being sedentary, this was not such a smart move. I thought I was going into cardiac arrest the first ten steps around that track! So I began walking while repeating a Bible verse I had read in a positive-thinking, mind-over-matter book: *I can do all things through Christ who strengthens me.*

Before long, I was able to run; and I've continued to run as a means of exercise ever since. With my recovery underway, it became apparent to me that I needed to seek emotional healing as well. I began to read any book I could find that would encourage me. I read nutrition and exercise books, as well as any recovery-type self-help books I could find. I even sought help from recovery programs for my drug addictions. Slowly, I began the process of rebuilding my life emotionally and physically.

Despite the progress I was making physically and emotionally, I found that I was still lacking peace and joy in my life. In all my reading I had not found one self-help, or step-by-step process book that could fill my empty heart. I had done all I knew to do to be healthy and joyful, but the void remained. In fact, I remember desperately fearing that I would die without ever knowing what it was like to experience true joy. During this searching period of self-recovery, my "religious" brother had many times told me that the void I felt in my life could only be filled by God. Over time I found myself agreeing with my brother, but the problem was, *How was I supposed to "get" God into my life?*

Answering that question became my focused pursuit. Out of desperate curiosity I began attending Sunday service at a church near the track where I ran. It was in that place that my spiritual journey began. Each week I drank in the sermon. Six weeks later at the pastor's invitation, I offered my life to Christ. I gave Him permission to take it and do whatever He wanted to do with it. (Before this decision point, I had only known of God—I didn't really know *who God was*.) That decision was the beginning of my spiritual healing; and on that day joy was born!

With God's help, I have rebuilt my life from the inside out. I have become what I truly believe is a "new creation." I no longer view my body as something to beat into submission and despise. Rather I realize I should honor God with my body and care for myself with love because He created me, loves me, and the Bible says I'm His temple. This totally transformed my life, because my heart was changed. I have joyfully come to believe that I'm His daughter and He loves me just as I am. I no longer have to turn to food or anything else to comfort me or ease any pain I may be experiencing.

Since the time of my "spiritual birthday" back in 1990, I have enjoyed my new life in so many ways. I have remained free from alcohol and drug addiction, and I've lost the extra 80 pounds of "me" I had been carrying around. Honestly, though, the road to my recovery from food addiction has not been perfect. I did have one setback when I became pregnant with my first daughter—gaining 60 pounds. But with the same knowledge and determination I had used to lose the weight the first time, I once again shed the weight. This time I have successfully maintained my healthy weight for over 16 years!

My life in my forties is characterized by healthy decisions, such as eating

healthy foods, exercising, sleeping well—and above all else, spending
time learning about and talking with God every day. As I give over my
life to Him, He gives me the ability to make the daily decisions that bring
stability, self-control, and enjoyment to the abundant life He promises.
I actually enjoy being healthy and exercising. I feel great; I have energy
for my family; and today I strive to model healthy living to my teenage
daughters. It is my hope that my girls will develop their own healthy self-
images and learn to love and accept who they are—despite the images
they are bombarded with through print and media. It is a challenging task,
but I know it must begin with me.

Chapter 7

Filling Your Heart Instead of Your Stomach

Emotional nourishment never gives you heartburn.

As you break free from your bondage to food, you will likely need "replacement therapy." Because food has long been your emotional "go-to," many of you will be heading off into this new, free world feeling somewhat empty and uncertain. Working through the last chapter taught you how to unload your emotional baggage—hence, your feeling of emptiness. Now you'll need to learn what to pack for a *healthy* life journey. This may leave you feeling somewhat uncertain.

If you empty out something and neglect to put something more worthwhile in its place, you'll find you end up filling it with junk again. At my house I like to think of it as the "garage principle." Every time my husband and I become disgusted as to how much junk is filling our garage, we—to be more accurate, *he*—set about emptying and reorganizing it. Then we stand back admiringly and proclaim how great it is to once again have order and space.

"Do you put one of your cars into that space?" you ask. No! We just let it stay vacant. But not for long…Empty space is a magnet for stuff! I don't care which side of the equator you live on. Likewise, if you empty your heart of painful emotions and don't purposefully replace that negative stuff with healthy alternatives, over time (usually sooner than later) you'll be overrun with emotional junk again. The healthy alternatives I'm talking about are assorted "heart-filling goodies" with which you bless yourself out of *love for yourself*—things such as self-care, self-respect, and self-control. This is why I call this chapter "Filling Your Heart Instead of Your Stomach."

Many of you may have forgotten what having a healthy relationship with food looks like. Some of you may *never* have had a healthy rapport with food. That's why we are here together in these final chapters— to retrain your knee-jerk reactions to life's stressors so food never gets that same stranglehold over you again! In order to fully achieve and maintain freedom from food addiction, you'll need to guard against the threats lurking around you that could cause you to slip down that slope into chronic overeating again, almost before you realize you are losing your footing.

The replacement therapy I'm suggesting needs to encompass three main areas: 1) your daily actions and reactions, 2) your thought life, and 3) your lifestyle. This chapter will work on that first area, your day-to-day actions and reactions, which—when healthy—can create fullness in your heart rather than in your stomach. In the chapter that follows we'll concentrate on taking control of your thought life (yes, this can actually be done!). Finally, in chapter 10, I will show you how to put into practice a positive, health-producing lifestyle.

FILLING YOUR HEART...

"This Is Dedicated to the One I Love"

I believe there are two basic motives why people would take good care of anything (including themselves). The first reason is because *they genuinely value that particular thing* (or their own self). The second motivation would be that, even though they may not personally place great value on that "thing" in their possession (or themselves for that matter), they understand that they are caring for something that has been *borrowed from someone else* who places immense value on it. In fact, that other party would be truly grieved to find that their beloved treasure has been misused or worse yet, destroyed while on loan.

Project this reasoning onto your own battle with self-care and preservation. In order to fulfill the first motive for self-care you *must* love yourself—and that also means you must *like* yourself. I'm not talking about some prideful, egocentric sort of love. I believe we can humbly appreciate who we are and who we've been created to be, and honor ourselves (and our Creator) by being devoted to the care and well-being of our physical bodies. Goodness knows the Lord is madly in love with you! The prophet Jeremiah reminds us,

> The Lord appeared to us in the past, saying: "I have loved you with an everlasting love; I have drawn you with loving-kindness" (Jeremiah 31:3).

Take your cues from the God of the universe, my friend—if He loves you, then you are most certainly lovable!

Here's the rub: Feelings follow actions. Even if you do not *feel* love for yourself, if you begin to *act* like you love yourself, psychology tells us that you will, indeed, begin to feel love for yourself! Quite amazing, isn't it? My pastor has encouraged our congregation more than once to "act ourselves into a feeling." I've tried it myself and have found that this method works surprisingly well. I am encouraging you to do the same. What have you got to lose—except a bunch of weight?

You may still be questioning the second motivating factor—the "borrowed body" suggestion. Who exactly is your body borrowed from? Well, the Bible holds the answer to that question. In 1 Corinthians 6:19-20 we read,

> Do you not know that your body is a temple of the Holy Spirit, who is in you, whom you have received from God? You are not your own; you were bought at a price. Therefore honor God with your body.

If you are a believer in the Lord Jesus Christ, your body is not yours to do with as you please. That being true, I urge you to take good care of that which has been loaned to you. This way, you'll be able to stand unashamed before your Maker when you return your earthly tent to Him at your life's end.

If you are married, you'll likely recall back on your wedding day the officiator of your marriage confirmed that indeed "the two have become one flesh." This implies that not only is your body on loan from God, but it also belongs, in part, to your spouse. What you choose to do with and to your body affects your marriage partner, both now and in the future. So demonstrate your love for yourself, your God, and your spouse by taking care of your body. If you can get these motivations to take up residence in your heart, then you'll find you've become one conscientious caregiver—and everyone will be the blessed!

Treat Yourself Right

People who care *about* themselves take care *of* themselves. This goes far beyond what you eat or don't eat. Let's drop a stone into the pond of healthy self-love and take note of some important ripples that extend out from the initial point. In my own life there are a number of things I do to "love on myself." Maybe a new lightbulb will go off for you and you'll follow suit.

Get Moving

One of the first ripples I see spreading across the pond of self-love is exercise—probably because I am a physical therapist. If you know it's good for you, you don't have to like it, just do it. It isn't necessary to join a gym or take Pilates classes. You can simply choose to move more...take a walk, ride a bike, or use an exercise DVD at home, anything! Twenty minutes, three to five times a week, is all it takes to love yourself through movement. And the benefits of exercise are felt throughout your body—even your brain, where "feel-good" chemicals are released as a result. These compounds can aid in combating depression and fatigue, giving you an overall sense of mental well-being. That's worth getting up off the couch for!

Dress for Success

Physical appearance typically demonstrates what a person thinks about themselves. What does your appearance say about you? Look at yourself in the mirror—do your clothes flatter your body (whatever shape you have), or do they hang from your body in an attempt to hide your flaws? Even overweight people look larger when their clothes are too loose-fitting. And keep your clothes sizes up-to-date with your weight loss. Don't spend all the effort to lose 20 pounds and then not reward yourself with a few new, well-fitting outfits— just because you still have another 20 pounds to go. Motivate (love) yourself along the way. It also helps others to become cheerleaders, rejoicing with you about your progress and encouraging more of the same. If you keep hidden under baggy clothes, your weight loss will remain your own little secret.

"Groomingdales"

Women, you will find it easier to love yourself if you feel put-together. (Don't you always admire those who do?) For some of you that may mean covering up the gray in your hair or adding a bit of makeup. Some women look beautiful with natural gray hair and clear complexions—but do you? If you don't know where to begin, recruit a fashionable friend. One of my friends has used me as her personal shopper from time to time. We started with the basics—undergarments. Sometimes women can use a lift, if you catch my drift!

Men, is your hair neatly combed? Did you shave this morning? Are you (look down) wearing black socks with shorts and sandals? (A fashion faux pas if you're unaware.) Are your clothes worn out or stained and in need of replacing? An outward appearance that says, *I care enough about myself to spend some time putting myself together this morning* speaks volumes to those around you. If you look like you don't care about yourself, how many people will feel drawn to care about you? Pursue looking your best out of *love for yourself,* because being well-groomed can lead to feeling good about yourself; which also lends itself to thinking great thoughts about who you are and what you can accomplish!

Rest

Everyone needs a little down time. You are no exception. Rest can take many forms. It could be drinking a cup of tea with your feet up for five minutes, taking a short work break or midday siesta, or allowing yourself a few uncluttered moments to take some deep breaths while daydreaming...but it must be about pleasant, nonworrisome things. One of the ways I show love and concern for myself in this area is that I make sure I get a good night's sleep (as far as I can control). That means I'm ready and in bed (lights off) 8 hours before I need to wake up the next day. Your body, mind, and soul will all be refreshed following a solid night's sleep. Guard yourself in this way from fatigue...which is proven to be one of the driving forces behind excessive hunger and overeating.

"Re-create-time" (Recreation)

We all need to have outlets built into our lives that bring pleasure, rejuvenate us, and provide us with some plain ol' sidesplitting fun! My many jobs and roles in life (author, professor, physical therapist, mother, wife, friend, and volunteer) require me to be highly productive most of the time. So in order to make sure I stay balanced emotionally, I schedule in a variety of self-enjoyment opportunities throughout my calendar week. When the weather is nice, I may go out by myself for a walk or a bike ride. If the weather is less agreeable I do enjoy going clothes shopping—what can I say, I'm a woman! Another thing I do is I schedule an "adult play date" with a friend each week. Sometimes I meet a friend for a meal, a cup of coffee (during which I usually drink tea), and sometimes we go for a walk on the boardwalk. Laughter and pleasure most certainly lighten our emotional loads. I am refreshed and encouraged by the time I spend with my friends. It truly feeds my soul! And speaking of feeding my soul...

Spiritual Food

Monday through Friday, before my workday begins I make sure I'm well-fed spiritually. For me that means spending quality (and quantity) time in prayer and Bible study. I find that when my heart is well fed, my other organs don't get so hungry! Sunday is, of course, my Sabbath. On that day I join my church's members in worship and enjoy feeding on my pastor's sermon. In the New Testament, Jesus quotes a passage from Deuteronomy: "Man does not live by bread alone, but by every word that comes from the mouth of God." (I knew my "quiet time" was somehow related to this whole food thing.) For some of you, eating spiritual food will prove to be a major appetite suppressant.

Life-Giving Relationships

Some of you may believe that you are an island. In your past, people you've invited to live with you or spend time on your island always brought pain with them. So you sent them sailing off and closed your borders to any other "life intruders." Possibly you are cordial enough to let others sail near your island, but you've sworn off intimate relationships—where you know and are known by another. It's not uncommon for people, especially those who have suffered emotional wounds resulting in addictive behaviors, to isolate themselves. Does isolating yourself from life-giving relationships sound healthy? I hope not. Let's look at what I consider to be a few people you would benefit from being around.

A True Friend

"A friend is someone who sticks closer than a brother"—or sister for that matter. (Paraphrased from Proverbs 18:24.) A true friend has your best interest in mind. They are not jealous of you or of the time you spend with another. They build you up and encourage you to be your best. Choose your friends wisely. Be on the lookout for someone who embodies the fine traits I mentioned. You have to sift through quite a bit of mud to come up with a diamond! But when you find one, you'll both be blessed to "do life together."

A Supportive Family Member

I qualified this one for a reason. Not all family members are supportive, even if their "title" would seem to require that trait. Gravitate toward the one or ones who extend grace to you, as they have surely had opportunity to see all your bad sides! Spend time talking to those who encourage you on this journey toward health and well-being. A loving supportive family member is worth their weight in gold—and at today's gold prices, that's an awful lot!

A Wise Counselor

Most of us need some professional counsel from time to time. This can be received from a respected psychologist or psychiatrist, or from a pastor or even a lay counselor. Some of you may need intense counsel, extending over many months. Others may need only a session or two just to "get your head screwed on straight." I know I have benefited throughout the years from occasionally going to speak with my pastor's wife, who heads the counseling ministry at my church. Sometimes you and I need to verbally work through an emotion with someone who is on the "outside" of that emotional setting.

Let me add one comment. If you are given wise counsel and fail to follow through with it, and your life spirals further down, don't go back just to "dump" on that counselor with no intention of taking the advice. You'll be wasting your time and theirs.

A Faithful Accountability Partner

"If one falls down, his friend can help him up. But pity the man who falls and has no one to help him up!" (Ecclesiastes 4:10). An accountability partner when dealing with addiction recovery is crucial. If you are involved in an organized weight-loss program, such as Overeaters Anonymous or First Place 4 Health, then you will be instructed to do exactly that. If you are trying to "go it alone" in weight loss and addiction recovery, please *don't.*" "Alone" equals failure time and time again. Set yourself up for victory. Find someone you can be accountable to. You'll be glad you did.

...NOT FILLING YOUR STOMACH

Name That Emotion

When I was a young girl, there was a popular television game show called *Name That Tune.* Players would win cash prizes by more quickly naming the title of a song that was "sung" (with la-la's) than their opponent. It took an attentive, practiced ear to recognize a popular song in just two or three "la-la" notes! These contestants must have spent years listening to songs and show tunes, over and over again, to become so adept at recognizing the tunes before a melody could even begin to be formed.

Here's my analogy. Become an expert recognizer—not of song tunes, but of your feelings. Be able to quickly recognize and "name your emotions." This will take some practice, but the more attention you pay to the "sound" of your emotions, the earlier you'll recognize them and be able to come out on top, instead of allowing your emotions to win that round. If you diligently practice your "Midbook Assignment," you'll be able to identify an emotional attack and, using the knowledge gained in the last chapter, defuse it before it can do you any damage. This tactic is much like the military's Patriot missile defense system, which uses radar to locate, identify, and destroy the incoming missile *before* it reaches its target. You and I need such a defense tactic if we are to avoid getting bombarded by the emotional stressors in our lives.

The Emotional 9-1-1

You've identified an emotional affront. What now? You should thoroughly reprocess that emotion using the guidelines given in the last chapter. But because life can come at you awfully fast sometimes, I want to give you a reference chart that can offer you a "quick emotional fix." But it requires acts of humility on your part. See if you're game.

Emotion	Your response
Resentment	Submit to authority
Guilt	Confession
Hurt feelings, bitterness	Forgiveness
Stressed out	Accept from God the things you cannot control
Anger	Willingly give up your rights
Fear	Trust in God as your protector
Worry	Have faith in the Lord regarding your future

Calming Your Trigger Finger

There are times when your past overeating behavior will raise its ugly head. There are overeating triggers that can send you speeding downhill. You'll need to identify and guard against these triggers in your own life. Certain types of food may just make you weak in the knees. What are they for you? Chocolate, doughnuts, pasta, potato chips, french fries? Do your best to not come face-to-face with them or bring them into your home. If you must be in the same room with such temptations, strengthen your resolve and walk away.

Social events can really do you in if you are not on the lookout. You would be wise to plan for a possible temptation attack beforehand. Do family holidays stress you out? Do you find yourself overeating just to tolerate the day? Maybe your mom makes the best desserts in West Texas...Whatever the situation, resolve to confront and control your desire to overeat, before you even lay eyes on all those scrumptious yummies! (For specifics on how to make this work, see chapter 9.) The same holds for true for parties, office get-togethers, and the like. Love yourself enough to control yourself. That's the bottom line.

Care for yourself,
Respect yourself,
Control yourself...
Ripples in the pond of self-love.

Chapter 8

You Are What You ~~Eat~~ Think

You can control what you think about.

The real battle to be waged against your overeating behavior does not take place between your mouth and your stomach. Rather it is fought between your ears. The way out of any addiction lifestyle begins in the deep recesses of your mind. What you think about, day in and day out, has a far greater impact on your future body weight than which diet method you end up choosing. As someone who has spent a significant amount of time in the overweight category, did any of your past weight loss efforts include a "thought diet"? Probably not. Society has programmed you to believe that weight loss is all about food restriction. I'd like to suggest that it is not. It is more about *thought* restriction.

Imagine if your private thoughts were able to be heard by those around you. If strangers and loved ones could listen in on your self-talk, I'm guessing you'd be more careful as to what you said to yourself—I know I would! Funny thing is, you and I talk to ourselves all day long (sometimes aloud), yet we rarely give a second thought as to the impact our self-talk is having on our own "ears." Don't allow yourself to be fooled, even if you're not consciously tuned in to your thought life—subconsciously you are! For this reason the content of your self-talk has a huge impact on the person you are today (condemned or inspired) and how successful you will be in the future at moving beyond the past and overcoming your present overeating addiction.

Seventeenth-century philosopher René Descartes, when contemplating a proof for the existence of man, declared, "Je pense donc je suis" (French), and later "Cogito, ergo sum" (Latin). Translated into English his statements read, "I think, therefore I am." What this philosopher was trying to "prove" was the idea that the conscious knowledge of producing our own thoughts provides us with the evidence that we in fact exist. Because I look at life's existence from a spiritual and scientific perspective, with all due respect I would reverse Descartes' statement. I believe it is more accurate to believe that: "I am, therefore I think." We are created, the Bible says, in God's own image. And God's mind is never idle! And, boy, have we humans been wired to think. Sometimes it seems our minds never rest—not even at night!

❧

Where do all our thoughts come from anyway? Psychologists tell us that most of our thoughts take root in our assumptions, or our held belief system about ourselves, the world around us, and our view of God. This is especially true of those thoughts which replay over and over again. Whether positive or negative, your thought life has tremendous influence on your life's course. Jennifer Rothschild, in her book *Self Talk, Soul Talk*, describes this effect well.

> The words we say [to ourselves] go straight to the core of our being. They shape the way we think about ourselves. They influence our emotions, our thoughts, and our decisions. They resurface in our conversations with other people. They can spur us on to live meaningful, productive lives, or they can drag us down to lethargy and despair.[1]

And overeating, I might add.

Psychologists have noted that many people struggling with food addiction are largely unaware of the one-sided conversations taking place in their heads throughout the day. (Sort of like a second-grade teacher who, by mid-year, barely notices the continuous chatter of her students.) Even when these pervasive thoughts go unacknowledged, they still are capable of holding you hostage under a heavy blanket of despair. Quite unannounced they can give rise to negative feelings which seem to come out of nowhere. Ever been ambushed by a strong emotion and wondered, *Hey, why am I suddenly feeling this way?* The fact is that when your head talk is negative, then you will *feel* downtrodden.

On the other hand, if you are engaged in positive self-talk, you will *feel* uplifted. This truth exists because we have been created in such a way that our feelings most habitually follow our thoughts. In order to get to the bottom of the unwanted emotions you experience (which are pressing you to reach for something to eat), you'll need to begin by prying into your own thought life. You must learn to recognize and purge the harmful thought data that up till now has been allowed free rein in your mind. The second thing you must learn how to redirect or replace is those ratty old thoughts with new, health-producing, life-giving ones.

Thus far, for ease of discussion, I have been overgeneralizing the thoughts you and I have as either *positive* or *negative*. Actually, self-talk more accurately falls into one of four distinct "thought categories."* As you read through the chart below, you'll notice I have separated thoughts which carry *a negative* message into two separate categories, *Type 1, Self-Accusation*, and *Type 2, Self-Evaluation*. The difference is, one message has a destructive outcome, whereas the other is productive. Likewise, I have divided *positive* self-talk messages into two other distinct categories, that of *Type 3, Self-Deception*, and *Type 4, Self-Inspiration*. Again, one of these self-declared messages has a destructive outcome, while the other is quite productive. In the sections that follow we'll take a closer look at these four distinct thought types so that you will be equipped to correctly judge and effectively control what it is you think about. If you are to win your battle against overeating, you must mentally police your mind. Some of your thoughts you'll find to be law-abiding, while others you'll have to apprehend quickly.

---

* Our minds also produce neutral thoughts, such as, *I need to put these letters in the mailbox* or, *It sure is warm outside today*. So that would make *five* categories, but I think I'll *choose* to ignore that last thought type!

The Four Types of Self-Talk

Type	Intended outcome	Nature	Message content	Reality	Influence on feelings, emotions, or behavior
1 Self-accusation	Destructive	Critical	Negative	False	Condemnation
2 Self-evaluation	Productive	Critical	Negative	True	Constructive
3 Self-deception	Destructive	Assuring	Positive	False	Denial
4 Self-inspiration	Productive	Assuring	Positive	True	Healthy

Type 1, Self-Accusation

This first type of self-talk is the major snare in the thought life of any addict. A self-accusing thought is a *critical, negative* message based in *falsehood*. Such a thought might be, *I will never be smart enough to measure up to my co-workers*. It will be followed by a chorus of other thoughts such as: *Your real problem is that you are lazy. And you never could understand things well. You can't do anything right.* These voices in your head relentlessly disgrace your person. They beat you up emotionally night and day—no wonder you feel like you do!

Self-accusing statements are generalized (non-specific) and begin with similar telltale banter:

- *I'm too*...stupid, boring, old, fat, poor.... for anyone to notice or care about me.

- *I'll never*...lose weight, be happy, smart, get a good job, finish my education, raise good kids, experience true friendship, have a healthy marriage.

- *I'm not*…important, attractive, funny, interesting, a good parent.
- *I can't*…do anything right, stick to a weight loss plan, get a promotion, be a good parent, run an organized home, understand my spouse.
- *I always*…make a mess of things, put my foot in my mouth, make bad decisions, fail.

Self-talk like this never points toward a specific corrective action or resolution. These thoughts are pure condemnation, through and through. Why do you keep telling yourself these hurtful things? Is it because someone else said them to you before and you are convinced they're true, or is it because of past failures you've had, or maybe it's because of your grim present circumstances? Whatever the cause, one thing is for sure. If you are going to step out of your addiction and into a world of freedom from overeating, the new you must come up with a different topic of conversation to engage in throughout your day! I'll show you how I do it in my own life as soon as we are finished identifying each thought type.

Type 2, Self-Evaluation

Thoughts which are self-convicting are also *critical* and *negative* in their message content. At first listen they may sound like a Type 1 thought; but listen more closely. What sets them apart from the thoughts we just discussed is that they are *spoken in truth*. Type 2, Self-Evaluation thoughts are actually your conscience calling you into *accountability and reform*. When one of these thoughts is brought to my own attention it might sound something like this: *Your were awfully harsh when you spoke to your son this morning.* How do I know that this statement holds truth? Well, two ways. First, if I honestly analyze the situation that occurred, I will find that the self-evaluation of my actions/attitude is, in fact, quite accurate (as much as I sometimes hate to admit it). And furthermore, if I ask an uninvolved party for their opinion, they will likely agree with my own evaluative self-criticism.

Secondly, these Type 2 thought-statements are *specific to a situation* such as *You shouldn't have yelled at your daughter when she accidentally knocked over that plant*. The purpose of a self-evaluating thought is to *confront us* and our actions, *not condemn us*—and that makes all the difference! When confronted with specific details, I am left with a choice of specific action which can have a productive outcome (if I follow through with it). In the case of my example, I can humble myself, apologize to my daughter, and seek to make things right between us. A condemning thought based on the same situation would sound more like this: *You can never control your tongue*—which would leave me accused without any specific way to redeem myself. If you are catching on so far, you would categorize that "useless" condemning thought as Type 1, or Self-Accusation.

Type 3, Self-Deception

Gee, now these thoughts sound very pleasing to the ear at first listen. They are not only *self-assuring* but they have a *positive* message as well—just what you want to hear, right? Wrong. These thoughts are lies, lies, lies. They exist primarily to create denial. *I am not a food addict*, you tell yourself. *I just like to eat*. Or...*I don't need any help losing weight. I'm just not ready to begin. I'll lose this weight when I'm good and ready, no problem*. Get the idea. This type of self-talk entices you down a pathway toward destruction, and all the while you're telling yourself you're on the road to Disney.

The Bible explains why knowing the truth is so critical to recovering from addiction. In John 8:32 we read: "You will know the truth, and *the truth will set you free*." Yes, my friend, that is the secret. If you can successfully identify, agree with, and hold onto the thoughts in your head that are true, you *will* be set free from overeating—and from all the other underlying emotional baggage that has kept you in your "fat clothes" for far too long!

Type 4, Self-Inspiration

Ahh, now these are the very best thoughts to entertain. Hey, they can stay all week if they'd like! These self-generated mental statements are *self-assuring, positive* and, even better, they are *true*! I like to think of this type of self-talk as nutritional food for your mind (and ultimately your heart, soul, and body as well). This is the type of thought life that sets a person up for success—as its outcome is always constructive. Self-inspiring self-talk boosts your self-image and provides the assurance and motivation you need to pursue change.

Remember, because these statements are based in *truth*, you need not fear that they will lead to pride. Pride comes from wallowing in Type 3, Deceptive self-talk, which can most certainly become boastful. In the same way in which you get to select what your body will dine on each day, you also get to select (for the most part) what your brain will feed upon. It really depends on what it is you put into the "shopping cart" of your mind. You can only cook up that which you have the ingredients for! Add to this healthy thought diet a measured dosage of Type 2, Self-Convicting thoughts as vitamins and you are on your way to a better, more vibrant you!

Now that you know what makes a thought either acceptable or unacceptable to entertain, it is time that you move on into your new roles as "destructive-thought apprehender" and "productive-thought encourager." Do you think you can do it? I'm certain you can. All you need is a little instruction.

The Conception of Your Thoughts

It is important that we recap the cascade of events that flow out from your personally held beliefs or assumptions. Your views on self, life, and the world around you (including your thoughts on God), are the basis for your private thought life—regardless of whether those views are true or false. Next, your thought life will undoubtedly give rise to your feelings (emotions). And just as "an apple does not fall far from the tree," your felt emotions will closely reflect your thought life. Because of this sequential process, destructive thoughts will yield negative, unhealthy feelings and constructive thoughts, positive, healthy feelings. The cascade further continues to overflow into the way you live your life. Those self-created feelings or emotions ultimately cause you to respond in like manner with characteristic actions, reactions, or inactions. In this way, your innermost thoughts and beliefs, which began as private, have now become apparent to all in your outward behavior. Your held beliefs have become your reality. To summarize,

$$\text{BELIEFS} \rightarrow \text{THOUGHTS} \rightarrow \text{FEELINGS} \left\{ \begin{array}{l} \rightarrow \text{ACTIONS} \\ \rightarrow \text{INACTIONS} \\ \rightarrow \text{REACTIONS} \end{array} \right.$$

Now let me give you a concrete example of what I am talking about:

Belief = *My birth was an "accident."* →

    Thought = *Nothing I do matters to anyone.* →

        Feeling = Worthless →

            Action = Overeat/binge

            Inaction = Don't care to groom yourself well

            Reaction = Distrust when someone compliments you

Isn't it remarkable how just one falsely held belief can bring about a whole cascade of grief! Now you can see why you must begin at the very beginning—altering your "mind's eye." Everyday conversational language speaks of a person's ability to practice self-imposed mind-control. Ever used any of these phrases?

"Have you *changed* your mind?"

"*Fix* your mind on it."

"You could if you *set* your mind to it."

"*Make* up your mind!"

"I can *call* to mind…"

Reread the words I emphasized. Each word is a verb, or a word which describes an action. By choosing to be an active participant in your own thought life, you can head off destructive thoughts and purposefully replace them with constructive ones. Practice is required.

But as with everything else in life, practice makes…no, not perfect, but very much improved!

How to Take Control

The Bible (my thought-life survival guide) contains verse after verse which agrees with the premise that you and I indeed have control over what takes up residence in our minds. In fact many of these passages are written as commands, rather than suggestions. The God who created us knew that any battle that would be fought with the body must first be waged in the mind. So He left us written instructions. I've listed some of these passages in the chart below for you. Alongside I have noted key portions of each passage that encourage you to take action against destructive thought patterns and *actively pursue productive ways of thinking.*

Scripture passage	What the Bible says you can do
Philippians 4:6-8 Do not be anxious about anything, but in everything, by prayer and petition, with thanksgiving, present your requests to God. And the peace of God, which transcends all understanding, will *guard your hearts and your minds* in Christ Jesus. Finally, brothers, whatever is true, whatever is noble, whatever is right, whatever is pure, whatever is lovely, whatever is admirable—if anything is excellent or praiseworthy—*think about such things.*	You can *guard* your heart and mind. You can *choose* what you think about.
Romans 12:2 Do not conform any longer to the pattern of this world, but *be transformed by the renewing of your mind.*	You can *renew* your mind.
Proverbs 3:21 Preserve *sound judgment* and discernment.	You can *obtain* good judgment. You can *practice* discernment.

Scripture passage	What the Bible says you can do
2 Corinthians 10:3-5 For though we live in the world; we do not wage war as the world does. The weapons we fight with are not the weapons of the world. On the contrary, they have divine power to *demolish strongholds*. We demolish arguments and every pretension that sets itself up against the knowledge of God, and *we take captive every thought* to make it obedient to Christ.	You can *break down* strongholds. You can *take* your thoughts captive.
Isaiah 26:3 You will keep in perfect peace him whose *mind is steadfast*, because he trusts in you.	You can firmly *purpose* your mind.
Ephesians 4:22-24 You were taught, with regard to your former way of life, to put off your old self, which is being corrupted by its deceitful desires; *to be made new in the attitude of your minds*; and to put on the new self, created to be like God in true righteousness and holiness.	You can *change* the attitude of your mind.

Whether you choose to look at it from a secular or from a biblical standpoint, the fact remains the same: You are absolutely capable of sizing up, interrupting, and redirecting your thought patterns.

A Reconception

"I have to be honest with you, Lisa—I have my doubts as to whether it's really possible for me to *change* what I think about." I have questioned the possibility as well. But I have experienced such victories in changing my mind on some very key issues, so much so that I am writing this chapter to testify that it most certainly can be done!

Case in point: I grew up with a very intelligent, very critical father who had earned himself a master's degree in English literature. Whenever I would ask him to read a paper I had written for school, be it a factual report or a creative writing piece, my self-esteem would take a beating. My father would tear my writing apart, tell me how awful it was, and laugh at my attempts to be creative.

What do you think my *held belief* was as I entered adulthood? That's right—"I can't write." The *thought* that followed was, *I should find a career that doesn't require writing.* How did I *feel* about my ability (or inability) to write? I was embarrassed (and definitely insecure) when it came to showing anyone anything I wrote. (Good thing I was a biology/ physical therapy major! My papers were only graded on content, not "literary correctness or creativity.")

My emotions of embarrassment and insecurity yielded the *action* of hiding my writing ability, the *inaction* of avoiding writing tasks, and the *reaction* of never accepting a compliment based on my writing ability. My thoughts were so set that even though I received A's on everything I had ever written and had a professional article published early on in my career which was published without revisions, I still heard myself say, "I can't write." And I didn't just say it to be humble, I meant it.

Imagine my dismay when in early 2006 God informed me it was time to write a book! *Not me, Lord! You know I can't write…*Well, this is my third book, and my first two books have needed little editorial intervention, I'm told.

In order to even attempt this task of writing books, I had to do some major refereeing of the thoughts that were in my brain, and I had to allow some new information to take up residence.

So how exactly can you bring about a similar change of mind for yourself? There are three sequential steps I used in order to properly filter through the thoughts that passed unchallenged through my mind day in and day out. As you try these for yourself, at first it is going to seem like panning for gold—a whole lot of mud and very little gold. But in the end you will find glimmering nuggets of truth that will be worth your effort. And you will have a much richer life! I know I do.

JOURNAL TIME

Step One: Becoming a Mind Reader

In your "Midbook Assignment" I asked you to note the emotions that you felt before and after you ate. Through that assignment many of you likely uncovered feelings you didn't even know were associated with your hunger. Now that we've determined that all those unwanted feelings begin as faulty thoughts, I'd like you to get out your journal again and begin to record some of the actual thoughts you "overhear" during the course of your day.

A good place to begin is with any Type 1, Self-Accusation, thoughts you catch wind of. If you find that when you mess something up during the day you exclaim, "Oh, I'm such a fool!"—write that down as one of your held beliefs. Or if you are getting yourself dressed in the morning and you mutter, "I can never look put together," write it down. These statements, and others like them, are birthed from your belief system.

Interestingly, I have found that when harmful self-talk like this is written out in black and white (exposing it to the light of day for truth analysis), it can be confronted directly and dealt with swiftly. As a result, it quickly begins to lose its hold on you.

I also would like you to keep a record of constructive thoughts you have as well for comparison. Remember, these thoughts don't always have to sound positive, but they are always based in truth. If you are diligent to record a few thoughts each day, soon you'll find that you have compiled a long list by the week's end. When you've got some thought material to work with, grab your journal and let's begin our interrogation. It will soon become apparent which thoughts are keepers and which ones should be thrown back.

Step Two: The Interrogation

Let's begin with the first thought on your list. Write out the thought at the top of a fresh page. Now see if you can come up with an answer for each of these questions below.

1. What is the source of this thought?
2. Where will this thought lead me if I continue to follow it?

3. Will it get me where I want to go?

4. Does it fit with who I am or where I wish to be?

5. Does this thought make me feel guilty, ashamed, angry, or fearful?

6. If I shared it with someone else who has an honest opinion of me, would they agree?

7. Does it fit with my statement of faith?*

8. Does it agree with biblical Scripture?*

Do you have enough information to determine whether that thought was destructive or if it can be released back into your thought pool (neutral or constructive)? Use this method of questioning with each of the thoughts you've recorded in your journal. Now, anytime you see the same thought (or a close cousin) hanging around your mind looking for trouble, you can automatically press the reject button, because you've already proven he's a bad guy! Since I've begun writing, I've had to be on heightened alert with regard to my *You can't write* thoughts. I did the work of determining they were based in error, on one man's opinion. All other opinions I've received since then are in conflict with my falsely held belief.

After you have gained experience using this line of interrogation from the outset of a thought, you will soon be able to quickly determine which thoughts can stay and which need to be placed under arrest. Quickly you will find that your mind just can't come up with anything new. All its old material just won't work on you anymore. It has no other choice than to generate something else more positive. (*You know what, I can write!*)

Step Three: Tell Yourself the Truth, the Whole Truth, and Nothing but the Truth...

...So help you God! Here is a great place to invite God into the equation. The influence of the Holy Spirit in my own life is the primary reason for the successes I've had in controlling what I think about. I daily utilized prayer to assist me in changing my mind. I urge you to

---

* See "In Christ" on page 172.

consider it for yourself. The Holy Spirit's power trumps willpower any day of the week! (See "Making My Story Yours" on page 177.)

Because I am sharply aware of the power that words have had in my own life, I was determined to raise my children with a keen awareness of it as well. When my son was much younger, he would from time to time, come crying to me to report something hurtful that had been said to him. I would purposefully respond by kneeling down to his level, looking him squarely in the eye, and asking him directly, "Well, is that the truth about you?" If it was determined that the hurtful name-calling was said merely as a mean-spirited barb, I would follow up by asking him to tell me what the real truth was about him. When he answered me with that truth, we agreed he should ignore the hurtful comment and hang onto the truth.

If, however, the statement held some truth (such as he was selfishly hogging toys), then I pointed out that what was said—even though it may not have been said nicely—did contain truth, nonetheless. I asked him to consider changing what he was doing or how he was acting so as not to provoke his playmate (typically his sister) to anger. In this way I enabled both my son and my daughter early on in their young lives to develop an analytical filter which could strain out Type 1, self-accusing thoughts or statements, yet allow Type 2, self-convicting thoughts and statements, access to their minds in order to, hopefully, bring about change in their behavior.

The example I gave was of a verbal scuffle. However, it displays exactly the same kind of processing you and I need to use when we hear ourselves making similar critical statements in our own minds. When we overhear self-talk that's critical or negative, we need to begin our own version of a lie detector test and ask ourselves a few pointed questions: *Is this thought warranted? Is there some truth to it? Should I apologize, repent, or change my behavior in any way?* Or is it, in fact, a big, ugly lie that needs to be taken out with yesterday's trash?

The Super Bowl playoffs just ended a few weeks ago. And while I am not a die-hard football fan, I always tune in for this last battle of the football season. Victory comes in the form of a well-conditioned, talented team of players who have practiced, over and over again, the plays in the coach's handbook. Without a well-rehearsed offensive and defensive plan, only defeat is in store. The same holds true for you and me. If we don't have a playbook for how we are going to deal with destructive thoughts ahead of time, we will get crushed by their opposition to our mental health. Study the play-by-play sequence listed below. Get really good at running it.

1. Carefully monitor the message being formed in your head.

2. As soon as you recognize the thought as untruthful, shut it down. Mentally slam the door on it. *Do not* invite it in for tea and discussion...

3. Replace it immediately with something positive and contradicting. (For example: *I can never finish my work on time!* can be effectively replaced with: *I have finished many work assignments on time. I will do my best to complete this one as well.*) Any positive statement declaring an opposing, truth-filled viewpoint will act as a silencer. It is sort of like "talking back to yourself"...without the stigma of disrespect.

   If you are a Christian, offering up praise to God is a very effective response to a "thought attack"—it downright frustrates Satan. Think about it; if his tempting thoughts trigger a reaction of praise for his arch enemy, Jesus Christ—you better believe he will stop the attack on your "mind-field." Recalling memorized Scripture addressing the specific negative thought also works well. (So for the example above: *I can never finish my work on time,* replace it with, *"I can do everything through him who gives me strength"*—Philippians 4:13.)

4. Make sure your mind stays out of trouble. It is, by nature, highly active. Keep it on a leash if you must. Give it plenty of healthy thoughts to feed on, safe places to run, and consistent discipline. In this way, you'll find it will grow to serve you—its master, well.

Be aware that current research studies find that it takes anywhere from 21 to 45 days to retrain a new behavior or to get rid of an unwanted habit. Destructive thinking is definitely a habit in need of breaking. So realize from the get-go that the intense part of this thinking boot camp will typically last for three to six weeks. Thereafter you will still need to be on guard for an occasional attack, but you will be serving during a time of peace, rather than during a time of warfare.

⊰◊⊱

Before we leave the subject of how to re-focus your thoughts, there is one other area I'd like to address—that of obsession. Realize that you are working through your obsession with overeating food. Don't replace it with another obsession! I have seen it happen to many people who have successfully lost weight through diet and exercise. Instead of living in freedom and self-control, they micromanage every morsel of food that goes into their mouths, weighing, measuring, counting... Their self-esteem rises and falls based upon whether or not they exercised that day. When you reach your realistic BMI (see chapter 1), live in the newness of your healthy lifestyle, but don't make it another weight to drag around with you for the rest of your days. We will talk further about what this looks like in the next chapter.

Danielle's Story of Hope

The first time I struggled with significant weight gain was during the summer following my high-school graduation. I had the exciting opportunity to travel with a music outreach team for four months. Since the majority of my days were spent sitting on a tour bus with nothing to do but eat the special snacks the hosts had sent my team off with, and with little or no time to be active, I found myself with a very limited wardrobe at the end of the tour—by that summer's end, only my "stretchy" clothes fit. When I returned home I discovered I had gained 32 pounds! This began my first experience with dieting.

During the next 20 years of my life, I fought those same 30-plus pounds, losing and gaining about 20 of them many times over. I could only manage to keep the weight off for about six months before starting to gain them back again. During this time I did give birth to four children, but I can honestly say that my pregnancies never caused a weight issue for me. I would always lose my extra "baby weight," returning to my prepregnancy weight within a few months after giving birth.

My problem was that my weight seemed to balloon *in between* having my kids (probably because I was using food to comfort myself from the everyday stresses of raising four little boys and ironically, at the same time I was battling boredom). Because I believed I could quickly lose my extra weight any time I wanted, I neglected doing anything—and ultimately found myself in a dangerous situation.

⟡

By the time I hit my late thirties the weight piled on at an alarming rate.

At 40 years old I weighed a dangerous 186 pounds. and wore a size 16! I had read the weight charts. At only 5 feet tall, I knew I was obese. I felt overwhelmed and out of control. Much of my time was spent nursing regretful feelings. My weight was beginning to cost me physically as well. I was suffering with extreme pain in my knees and hips, skin irritations, and I was frequently sick. Yet knowing the focus it took to start and stick to a "diet" I used my lack of time as an excuse *not* to lose weight. Hey, I was far too busy working and being mom and wife.

However, my full schedule didn't stop me from thinking (obsessively so) about my condition. I spent every moment I could spare staring at calendars and calculating how much I could weigh by a certain date if I were to start a diet now—while at the same time regretting that I hadn't done so already. I found my thoughts were either focused on escaping to an imaginary future which included a skinny version of me, or dwelling on my disappointing past, where I mercilessly condemned myself. I began to realize that by spending so much time imagining the future or dwelling on the past, I was failing to address what was actually happening now—in real time. It was this realization that God used to start me on the road toward dealing with this issue in my life.

I began a personal relationship with God at a young age, and while I have enjoyed many blessings of walking closely with Him ever since, I had never really surrendered my eating and exercise habits to Him. I never accepted the fact that I was using food just as addictively as any alcoholic or drug user. Four years ago as we were facing some life-changing choices as a family, I had purposed to spend more time asking God for direction. As I searched His Word for answers and prayed earnestly for His counsel, a thought occurred to me that I knew immediately was not my own: My food addiction and my lack of focus on the here-and-now were hindering my ability to hear God speak.

It was no easy task to change my thought life—I had worn a very familiar path directly to *what life would be like if...* in my mind. Focusing my thoughts on the reality of the moment was unfamiliar territory. I felt lost, but, in my heart, I knew God was with me. At that time I recalled something my pastor had said in a sermon: "Do what you know you should do and then you will know what you should do." I knew immediately what that meant for me. God wanted me to do what I knew to do: give up the way I had been eating and treating my body. Yet I sensed He wanted more than just a decision to diet, He wanted a complete change in my thought life and in my desires.

This was actually an emotionally painful thing for me to do. My fantasy thoughts and I had become such close friends—and so had cookies! Yet I knew God wanted me to "take every thought captive." And since my every thought at the time was centered on food and the condition of my body, if I wanted to be obedient to God's Word, I had to stop my wishful or condemning thinking in its tracks and replace them with something else. Strangely, in addition to giving up my desire for sugary snack foods, I felt I had to give up my obsessive desire to be thin as well.

For me, letting go of my fruitless thoughts and desires felt like going through a grieving process. I guess this is what Scripture means when it asks us to "die to ourselves" and to live for Christ. Once I made this change however, I found God to be His usual faithful self. As I gave up my damaged thoughts He replaced them with His perfect ones. He gave me a new understanding that living for the satisfaction of only one part of my body (my mouth) was unholy and that living that way kept me from desiring more of Him. Now every time I was faced with an unhealthy choice, God was there to remind me of my new desire. I actually sensed Him saying to me, "I will still love you if you choose that, but will it get you what you want?" The obvious answer kept me focused.

⚜

Four years ago I began a new lifestyle where I only ate foods that would benefit my body, I walked for at least half an hour every day (while spiritually exercising at the same time through prayer and worship), and I purposed to think about gaining a greater sense of God's presence instead of focusing on losing weight. The change was far beyond anything I had ever wasted time dreaming about. Because my knee and hip pain was gone, my walking, which was very difficult at first to even continue for half an hour, gradually transitioned into a one-hour jog. Within nine months

I had a new body to match my new mind-set. I had lost 78 pounds and had dropped from a size 16 to a size 2!

I did have a brief setback three years ago after reaching "the goal I had never set." I indulged in a few of my old food choices thinking I could handle it—and alarmingly I gained 10 pounds in less than two weeks! But I experienced God's grace firsthand as He guided this foolish lamb (that would be me) back to within the safe boundaries He had enabled me to set in the first place (*Stay away from cookies!*). I lost those 10 pounds and haven't seen them again since. Even though I have reached a healthy weight, I consider myself to still be on a journey when it comes to controlling my thoughts, desires, and food intake. I now know that it would be foolish to believe that I could remain consistently on this road without God's help.

For the past three years I am happy to report that I am still a size 2 (the textbook size for my height and frame). I continue to run four to five days a week, covering 6 miles during each one hour run. Oh, and I haven't been sick in almost three years now.

Chapter 9

Best-Laid Plans...
Dealing with Setbacks

Shame is no longer the name of the game!

I must confess...I am a recovering plan-a-holic! Raised in a chaotic, reactionary home fashioned me to pursue this planning behavior full force. I had become fearful of the unexpected events in life (many which *should* have been planned for), which had created some very stressful times for my family growing up. So I was determined to minimize the times in which I was caught off guard.

During my twenties, however, I came to realize that planning *everything* didn't leave room for the unexpected, *fun* things in life. My existence lacked the "S" word...*spontaneity*. Also I realized that when taken to the extreme, my careful planning often left God's plans for my days unacknowledged.

Over the last two decades of my life I've slowly adjusted my ways and released my fear-driven planning grip over my future (as if I ever really had it under my control in the first place). What remains today, I believe, is a healthy propensity toward planning. I still plan my daily schedules (but now I give God full allowance to change them any which way He chooses), my family's weekly dinner menu, my household's annual and monthly budget, our vacations, and so on. Because of this responsible forethought, when faced with something *I already knew* was going to occur, I can be prepared, having already thought it through. No panic—I have a plan in place.

What I am suggesting is that you become a responsible planner yourself. Decide ahead of time how you will respond to your weight loss setbacks—before they occur. Listen to me, my friend, *there will be*, without a doubt, *setbacks*—no ifs, ands, or buts about it! To believe otherwise will surely set you up for future disaster.

My psychotherapist friend Scott Forsmith told me that there is a major issue of denial which accompanies the recovering addict, whatever their addictive agent was (is). He said that his patients commonly have a euphoric sense of victory over their successful recovery from their addictions. Unfortunately, many of his patients naively believe that once their addiction has been brought under control, they are completely immune to its re-entry into their lives.

Sadly, most of these patients end up struggling with relapses into their addiction behaviors, having convinced themselves that their mastery of their addictive agent was a "done deal." George Ohlschlager, JD, the senior editor of *Christian Counseling Today* magazine, wrote a biographical article entitled "A Personal Journey with Addiction." When speaking of his past drug addiction he admits that "even today, at the age of 56, I must guard against their siren call to relapse and use [drugs] again."[1] Dr. Ohlschlager has earned a doctorate in law, a master's in social work, and is a board-certified professional Christian counselor—still, by his own admission, has relapsed into drug use (once, in his thirties) and acknowledges that even today, 20 years later, he continues to feel temptation's pull toward his past addictive agent. Do *you* think you'll be better able to withstand such a temptation when it comes to food?

Let me explain why prematurely believing your overeating problem is "a thing of the past" can be dangerous and faulty. Most other addictive agents can be avoided. You have to go out of your way to wind up in a gambling casino. Drugs and alcohol can be purged from your home, and you needn't return to socializing at the bar or hanging around with those you used to get high with. Pornography can be resisted by setting up blocking software on the computer and avoiding risqué magazine racks. But you will never be able to avoid food. It is everywhere you go, at every function, in every restaurant, and at every sporting event. No matter where you turn, it's there—and you must keep some in your home. Because you have to eat to live, your addiction lends you countless opportunities to fall off the wagon—and into the potato salad!

You have come such a long way through the reading of this book. Hopefully, you have worked through some deep emotional pain, and I trust you are on the road to a healthy relationship with food. All I am saying is this: Don't put this book down prematurely; *be prepared for a setback*. Or as Dr. Hemfelt informed his patient in the book *Love Hunger*, "Dealing with relapse is *part* of your recovery program."[2]

The Warning Signs of Relapse

I have been evaluating and treating patients as a physical therapist for 20 years now. My postgraduate training as well as the practice settings I've chosen to work in has equipped me to specialize in the field of orthopedics. As a professor, I educate doctorate physical therapy students on the specifics of evaluation and treatment of patients with problems relating to their spine. My many years of experience have often enabled me to understand exactly what is wrong with my new patients before I even begin their physical evaluation—simply by asking them a few seemingly unrelated questions. This is because time spent in this field has allowed me to gain a sharp awareness of the "warning signs" of particular physical diagnoses and diseases.

Likewise, I want you to develop a similar alertness as to the warning signs of a possible relapse into food addiction. The more watchful you are, the quicker you will be at recognizing trouble brewing on the horizon and take preventive action. Keep the following *five warning signs* in the forefront of your mind so that if—or should I say *when*—any of them begin to surface, you can deal quickly and successfully with them before they upset the whole applecart.

Simmering Negative Emotions

Often after having done the big work of emotional recovery you will have the sense, *Hey, I'm over that feeling*—when in actuality, what you are really "over" is the situation(s) that created that destructive emotion. Your recovery work has brought closure to a past event.

But life goes on. We will always be susceptible to the reoccurrence of those same negative emotions. Maybe your parent recently shamed you by something they said. Perhaps your spouse or your boss at work blew up at you. Or possibly you've encountered a fresh new wave of *self*-abuse. *I'll never be able to stay thin. Nothing better is going to happen in my life because of all the weight I lost anyway…*You get the picture. Be in the habit of taking your emotional temperature from time to time. The best time to fight an emotional relapse is in its infancy, before it begins to present its grand demands: "I *need* chocolate cake!"

Denying the Truth

Eavesdrop on your own self-talk from time to time. You'd be surprised at the conversation you hear resurface. We are quite capable of misleading ourselves. Truth turns into lies when the truth is not cultivated, just like a patch of garden becomes overrun by weeds when the gardener is preoccupied with other things. Be alert to anything that sounds similar to these statements:

> I don't *need* to have any outside support anymore…
>
> My family relationships aren't actually *that* bad…
>
> I don't think I actually had a food *addiction*…
>
> You know, I wasn't really *that* overweight back then…

These statements are proof that truth has not been continually cultivated and denial has sprung roots. Weed out denial immediately, before it has a chance to grow.

Distancing Yourself from Support

When you are drowning in a sea of addiction, you are eager to scramble toward any life preserver that has been thrown to you. We spoke previously about the importance of a life-preserving human support/accountability system. For you, assistance may have come in the form of a friend, a support group, a counselor, or a pastor. But once you have been pulled to safety you begin to forget about the dangerous sea from which you were rescued.

Then one week you think, *I don't have time to go to those meetings anymore*...and you never return. You don't return the phone calls of your accountability partner—or at least you don't return them in a timely manner, so that maybe they'll get the hint that you don't *need* them anymore. Believe me, I am not suggesting that you keep up the rigors of recovery forever. I'm just reminding you to stay connected to someone who can keep you on their radar; someone you can rely on to keep you accountable when it comes to your ongoing relationship with food.

Flirting with Food

You are in Costco or Barnes & Noble one day and you suddenly feel drawn to the cookbook section. You thumb through the glossy pages, mouth watering and eyes lusting at the sight of all those forbidden delicacies. Your mind drifts back to "happier times" when you used to go to that all-you-can-eat buffet restaurant...*Man, their dessert selection was to die for...*

Excuse me—may I interrupt this trip down memory lane for just a moment? We've already established that no food is worth *dying* for. When someone is nearing a food abuse relapse they will usually begin "flirting" with food. Flirting always begins in the mind before it is expressed through an action. That means your "innocent" decision to stop by the bakery "to buy just one cookie" (flirtation) can quickly unravel into a full-blown affair! So if you find yourself thinking an awful lot about food, flipping through gourmet magazines for new dessert recipes, or purchasing cookbooks on impulse...well, you might very well be headed off the road.

Your Pants Are Too Tight

Been avoiding the scale? The fit of your clothes will keep you honest. And no, they didn't suddenly shrink in the dryer. If you monitor your weight weekly, you'll know when you have begun to slip down the slope into overeating. Weight gain of more than seven to ten pounds should be a red flag. There's no doubt that you have been cutting yourself some slack along the way. Maybe you've been increasing your portion size, or snacking after dinner. Have you been skipping your date with your treadmill or canceling out on your walking buddy? Or possibly you've begun feeling sorry for yourself (under such heavy food restrictions, and all)—so you've been treating yourself to a dish of ice cream or small bag of potato chips each night while you watch TV. Of all the warning signs, weight gain is the one that can't be denied. The scale, the mirror, and your clothes—they don't lie!

Each year the winning team of the Super Bowl loses some ground (yardage) throughout the game. Yet they always keep their minds fixed on the goal, push through the opposition, and as a result, advance to victory in the end. Please my friend, don't back down when faced with setbacks. Strengthen your resolve. The game is not over. Victory can still be had.

What to Do When It Happens to You

Health is a *journey*, not a destination. The road toward better health (which includes weight loss and maintenance of such) is paved with many potholes. Some of these depressions are shallow and merely set you off course a bit. (You had *two* servings of cake at a friend's birthday party last night.) Other ruts are deeper, causing you to veer off center a ways. (You go on a cruise vacation and eat everything in sight for a week.) Still other potholes are the pits—literally and figuratively. Sometimes, when you least expect it, along comes one of these pits, and down you go...and up your weight goes! Before you know it your weight is miles from where you want to be.

When one or more of these scenarios *does* occur, and you lose your way (and gain some weight), what will be your response? If you are still held in the grips of your past, you will likely hammer yourself with shame. Don't do it! Fight the urge to beat yourself up verbally and mentally. Rehearse in advance a different message to tell yourself. First, remember from where you came (allow yourself to feel proud about what you have accomplished overall), and second, assure yourself that you are capable of rising up out of that ditch once again and moving forward (give yourself a dose of hope).

The next important step toward resuming a healthy lifestyle is to make up with yourself—that's right, forgive yourself. Don't keep a laundry list of all the times you've slipped down into those same potholes and veered away from your goal of better health. Admit your guilt—say, "I forgive me," warn yourself, "Try not to let that happen again," and then move on. But recognize if it does happen again, you will need to encourage and forgive yourself all over again. How many times? I think Jesus mentioned something about seventy times seven...

Moving Forward

I love the saying "Deal with it, and be done with it!" It holds the sense of responsive action followed by forward, rather than backward looking. It settles the unpleasant occurrence with firm closure. That is what you desperately need to recover from a time of setback—regardless of how short or long it was—solid, undeniable closure. When exactly do you pull your life out of the pit of rebound? *Immediately.* As soon as you acknowledge you have slipped up, you must get back on track. The worst thing you can do is say to yourself, *Wow, I really blew that meal. I can't believe I ate the whole stack of pancakes, and my entire omelet! Well, this day is blown. I'll guess I'll start fresh in the morning.*

No! Every calorie you consume during the remainder of that day is another calorie you'll likely store as fat. Stop at once and turn your "car" away from the slippery slope of food addiction. The more time you spend spinning your wheels in that pit, the harder it will be to get yourself out. Remember, food does not have control over you—you have control over it.

Another important measure to take when recovering from weight-gain setbacks is to once again engage your communication with your accountability partner or group. You may have allowed that aspect of your life slide because you were doing so well. But you're not anymore, so get back in touch with the person, group, or organization who aided your success in the first place.

Life can be tough. We *all* need support along the way. Don't feel humiliated to return to something you thought you "graduated from." You don't feel embarrassed to take antibiotics each time you become sick with an infection, or to return to the service station when your car breaks down again, right? So why, when your overeating behavior starts to rear its ugly head, do you hesitate to seek accountability support again? It is often the only way back to wellness. Do yourself a favor. Make the call. Time's a-wastin'. And all those extra calories you've been eating—they're a-*waist*-ing!

My final recommendation is that you return to your formerly successful methods of losing weight. Run an inventory of where you are today and what you are presently doing (or not doing) and change course where need be. Hey, if the old way worked, why mess with it?

Maybe you need to go back to the journaling assignments as new situations and emotions may have recently surfaced. Possibly you have let your guard down when it comes to your food intake or have been skipping your exercise routine...whatever you recognize as part of the problem, resolve to restore "law and order" once again.

Lastly, this thought bears repeating: There should be *no shame* in setbacks, only guilt. And guilt is necessary to lead you to repentance and to give you the determination to do things differently going forward. Remember, relapse will likely be a part of your recovery process. Don't be overconfident. It is highly unusual to experience a perfectly paved road on your journey toward recovery from food addiction. If and when you do encounter a setback along the way, remind yourself of this Japanese proverb: *Fall down seven times, get up eight.* You can do it—I know you can.

Chapter 10

Presenting...the New You!

Food is no longer your master.

As you begin taking your first new steps in the land of freedom from food addiction, having spent so much of your time in the land of food obsession, you probably have little idea of what having a healthy relationship with food even looks like. What does it take to become a truly well-balanced person, one who can enjoy food without guilt and who has so many other interests and goals that food holds only its rightful place in the day—that of nourishment and pleasure, not a tranquilizer, Band-Aid, or time-filler? There are a number of features in your day-to-day world that will need to be polished up and returned to a prominent place on the mantelpiece of your life. When you're finished putting these tips for successful, healthy living into practice, you'll barely recognize your old self...and that's a good thing!

Food = Fuel

When I was a teenager my youth-group leader was married to a peculiar sort of man. Whenever you greeted Marvin, a dear soul, by asking, "How are you?" he always responded in the same way: "Happy, healthy, and thankful!" Being an engineer by trade, Marvin took the food equals fuel concept to a nuts-and-bolts level. Among other eating oddities, he was known to take a bag of peas out of the freezer and pop a handful into his mouth still frozen—because he had missed having a vegetable serving with his last meal! I'm not suggesting this type of detachment from the joy of eating. But the idea that Marvin fully grasped, and the one you can begin to digest, is this: Foods can refuel and recharge your physical body. That's the primary reason we eat—to fuel up for what lies ahead. (Marvin passed away on the very same day I wrote this, having lived 85 happy, healthy, and thankful years. May we all be so blessed!)

As with gasoline, there are different "grades" of food-based fuel. *Whole foods* (those that resemble their naturally grown or raised state) are typically best. The more processed a food becomes (bleached flour, white rice) and the more unnaturally occurring things that are added to it (partially hydrogenated soybean oil, high-fructose corn syrup, food coloring), the worse it becomes for you. A healthy relationship with food can be compared to a healthy friendship. Both partners need to gain from their relationship. (In the science world we call that a symbiotic relationship.) If one person continually harms the other, the relationship is an unhealthy one. It's best that an unbalanced partnership not be pursued. Instead pursue foods that promote your health, rather than leave your body in jeopardy.

Because food is fuel, you need to make sure your tank's gauge does not fall to empty. Here's how I, and others like me, stay trim: I *eat*! That's right. I eat a large breakfast each morning, followed by a mid-morning snack (maybe a handful of almonds). Later I eat a moderately sized lunch, another snack in the afternoon (like a piece of low-fat cheese or half an avocado), and finally I finish off the day with a healthy, home-cooked dinner. If I am hungry later on, I use extreme caution as to what and how much I eat. Usually I take one cookie or a square of dark chocolate from a bag, close it up, and walk away to eat it. (Never, never take the bag with you! The calories you eat in the evening will likely not get burned off, but rather stored away...so eat responsibly.)

Sense-ible Eating

Eating can be one of life's greatest pleasures. When God created us, He crafted us with five senses: sight, touch, hearing, smell, and taste. All of these senses add pleasure to what we eat. We were created to enjoy food, and food was created to be enjoyable. Fine restaurants know that your eating satisfaction is enhanced by artful food presentation. Cinnabon is quite certain we'll follow our noses through the mall to get to their cinnamon delights. And that crunching sound a fresh apple, some crusty bread, or a handful of chips makes when you bite into them can't be beat!

As for the sense of touch, your tongue is one of the most sensitive parts of your body—there are over 200 nerve endings per square centimeter on the tongue,[1] each capable of relaying messages to your brain about how smooth your yogurt is or how rough and pointy that granola you're munching on is. Someone who's in control of their eating can enjoy their food with all of their five senses but not become addicted to it. Much like a person who can enjoy a glass of red wine with dinner, fully appreciating its ruby color, floral bouquet, and full-bodied flavor, yet not seek to have another glassful and then another.

So by all means, enjoy what you eat—involve all your senses. Prepare your food to look, taste, and smell pleasing. And then, when you're finished with your healthy-sized portion, you'll walk away satisfied.

Correcting Portion Distortion

Researcher and registered dietician Jim Painter, PhD, RD, says, "Most of us eat whatever's on our plate." In one study he conducted, people who unknowingly ate soup out of self-refilling bowls consumed 73 percent more than those who were given regular bowls. "They just wanted to get to the bottom,"[2] he reports. Another study by Painter's research group showed that people who ate ice cream out of larger bowls with larger spoons ate a far greater amount of ice cream than their counterparts who ate out of smaller bowls with smaller spoons.[3]

Portion size is so important that it appears to even trump food *type*. In his documentary "Portion Size Me," Painter placed two of his students on a 30-day fast-food "diet." Eating only what was given to them (proper portion sizes), both students actually lost weight! Now, let me quickly say that I'm not validating continual fast-food consumption as a part of a healthy lifestyle. But I think Dr. Painter's findings drive home the point. Weight loss and maintenance are tied directly into portion control.

Because, as we know, too much of a good thing can become a bad thing, here are some of my tips you can use to improve your portion control:

1. When serving yourself, take a smaller amount than usual, and then put away the leftovers *before* you begin to eat. (It's risky business to bring the "extras" to the table. It takes 20 minutes for your brain to get the message that your hunger has been satisfied.)

2. Know visually what a healthy-sized portion should look like:

   - A one-cup serving of rice or mashed potatoes = the size of a tennis ball
   - One portion of meat = the size of your palm; it's about as thick as your index finger
   - A serving of vegetables fits inside your two cupped hands
   - One serving of fruit = the size of your fist, and so on...

3. Don't eat out of containers. You have no idea how much you are eating, and the temptation to overeat is often overpowering!

4. Check label for portion sizes and calorie counts when eating prepared, prepackaged foods.

5. When ordering in a restaurant:

   - Send the bread basket back! If you love bread (or are famished!), take a small piece of bread with some butter or, better yet, olive oil, and *then* send the rest of it away. (Adding the fat here in moderation satisfies your hunger and controls your blood sugar better than bread alone.)
   - Eat only half of your meal and "doggy bag" the rest. (If you don't have the willpower to stop halfway through, ask your waiter to package half of it *before* you begin.)
   - Order an appetizer and a salad instead of an entree.
   - If you absolutely must indulge, *share* a dessert.

A New View on Food

Finally, I'd like to suggest something that is sort of countercultural. *Avoid using food as a reward or a "consolation prize."* For many of you it began when you were young. (You may even be passing this type of eating behavior onto your children.) You brought home a stellar report card—so your parents took you out for a "reward milkshake." You performed with the school band on concert night, so your family went out to a fast-food restaurant to celebrate a job well done. Your soccer team won (or lost), so… "Let's all go get ice cream!" Your parents used food this way, other parents around you do as well, and so you continue doing what you know, conforming to what's culturally the norm.

If food is the only way to say "congratulations" or console yourself (or your child) after a disappointment or loss, then it easily becomes an unhealthy outlet for your emotions later on in life. My suggestion is, steer away from this possibly addiction-driving use of food. I'm certain you can discover new ways to deal with the emotional highs and lows of your family members. Think of other things or experiences that bring pleasure besides food. Try rewarding or consoling yourself (or your family members) with these alternatives: How about a picturesque walk, a trip to a craft or hardware store, or a ride to a bookstore to purchase an interesting book or magazine? Any of these can be done spontaneously.

With my own children I've used alternate means to celebrate events, such as sincere words of compliment or affirmation (spoken with direct eye contact and followed by a hug or a proud pat on their back) or the purchase of a nonfood treat (typically a clothing or music purchase for my daughter and a sporting goods something-or-other for my son). For times of disappointment, I give my downcast child time and attention to vent their frustrations. Then I add some of my own life experience and wisdom to help bring perspective to their loss. I never "feed away" their pain.

I'm not suggesting you *never* celebrate with food, but mix it up so that food is one of many celebratory treats. However, I would never use food to soften a hard blow or disappointment—that's just asking for trouble with food abuse.

Market Strategies

Much of your success in living as the new you can be undermined at the supermarket. For this reason, I've discovered the need to prepare for my own food shopping trips by employing some "market strategies." The first tip for success is sort of a no-brainer (as my kids would say): *Don't go food shopping when you're hungry.* If you must go on your way home from work, plan ahead and leave an apple or something in your car so you can fill your stomach first instead of filling your cart with not-so-good-for-you impulse buys. No one thinks clearly on an empty stomach.

Here's another important shopping tip: *Read the labels.* Pay attention to serving size and calorie count, saturated fat grams and fiber content. Then read the ingredients. You'd be surprised how many bad things are added to seemingly good food items. Case in point: Many whole-grain breads contain high-fructose corn syrup. And here's a specific example: I recently bought a box of "fiber fortified" granola bars for my kids. I did a quick scan of the label. Low sugar, no saturated fat, high fiber—great! I threw it in my cart. After my kids had finished the box, on the way to the garbage pail I glanced at the list of ingredients...*ugh—partially hydrogenated soybean oil. Drats!*

My final piece of marketing advice is this: *Buy foods you have to prepare and cook yourself.* Make the time to prepare your own meals—even if it has to become a weekend family activity. Take pizza as one example. If you purchase some uncooked dough at your local pizzeria, you can top it with some leftover homemade sauce, reduced-fat mozzarella cheese, and leftover cooked vegetables (my favorite is broccoli rabe). This way, not only do you save money, but you save fat grams and salt overexposure!

Soups and stews are other great home-cooked meal ideas. You can de-fat a soup or stew before you eat it by refrigerating it overnight and lifting off the unwanted fat that hardens on its surface. This gives you a healthy meal without all the fat, not to mention all the added salt and MSG found in the canned or prepackaged varieties. Keep in mind that unfortunately most everything "quick and easy" you bring home is filled with nutritional shortcuts as well. Be good to yourself and to your family—eat quality fuel.

Adding "New Moves" to Your Repertoire

How many people out there love to exercise? Can you speak up?… Just like I thought—not many. Myself, I love to do anything that involves other people. This obviously does not apply to waiting in long lines or riding a cramped NYC subway, but it pretty much holds true for me with regard to exercise. So an aerobics class or a tennis game, a walk with a friend, or a bike ride with my family…well, I'm all for that. But when I have to get on my treadmill five days a week (during the cold of winter) or take a solo bike ride—that's when I feel "internal resistance." But I make up my mind once and for all days that I will pursue health as best I'm able. Now that you've gotten free from emotional overeating, you also can make this kind of decision.

The simple key to weight reduction and then weight maintenance is, don't let the calories that go in become greater in number than the calories that go out (or are burned up). Not only does exercise use up calories (even after you are finished sweating), but it also increases your metabolism, improves your mental state, and decreases your risk for many diseases. Exercise in some way, shape or form, really is a non-negotiable for the new you!

Mirror, Mirror on the Wall…

Once you begin to lose a significant amount of weight, you will need to change your wardrobe. As you downsize your clothes, there's one thing you need to up-size: the appreciation you have for your body. The new you needs to be at peace with the image your mirror is reflecting back at you. Few in this world ever look into a mirror with complete satisfaction—that includes supermodels! Yet, while you have the understanding that not everything looks the way you'd wish, accept yourself for who you are. *This is the "me" I've been given. How can I make the best of it?*

Also, every healthy person needs to have a reasonable weight-target range to work toward and maintain. (Refer to the BMI calculator in the "Resources for Healthy Living.") And "not for nothing" (as some people from Brooklyn put it), you need to understand and accept that your Creator made you with the body size, type, skin color, and ethnicity He wanted for you. To argue with Him about the results of His creation would be ungrateful and disrespectful. Further, it primes you to jump back onto the food-addiction cycle. Make peace with who you are, on the inside and on the outside. Trust God—His Word says you were made with a particular form and function (Jeremiah 1:5; Ephesians 2:10). When you do, your days will be filled with purpose, and your nights with peace.

A *Friend*-ly Reminder

The new life you are seeking to embrace includes embracing others. As we already discussed, when you are overweight or obese you tend to limit the number of people you interact with. Even more telling is that the number of people you actually "get real with" are far fewer. If you're going to live a healthy existence, that existence must include meaningful, safe relationships.

Now, some siblings are very close, almost surpassing the need for a "bosom buddy." While that may be the case for you, I do encourage you to find at least one person outside of your marriage or family of origin to become close with. Life holds far too much drama to place all the burden of your emotional support on only your spouse and one other person. The new you needs a variety of people to "do life" with. (That said, I don't believe you should seek a close friendship with a member of the opposite sex—especially if you're married. It can really mess things up for you emotionally in the long run.) Anyway, if you're no longer going to use food for comfort, you'll need to find some "safe" friends who are willing to take on that much needed job description.

Though everyone understands what a *meaningful* relationship is, some of you may be confused over this relationship needing to be *safe*. For a quick way to know if a relationship is safe, use this list:

> A safe friend is...
>
> ...kind, thoughtful, not jealous of you or the time you spend with another friend. Their words build you up, and they are honest, trustworthy, and self-sacrificing for your friendship (you don't always have to do things their way). They're not easily angered, don't keep a laundry list of your shortcomings, and they always want to see you succeed!

The Bible paints a beautiful word picture of friendship. In Ecclesiastes 4:9-10, the writer, King Solomon, proclaims,

> Two are better than one, because they have a good return for their work: If one falls down, his friend can help him up. But pity the man who falls and has no one to help him up!

That is the beauty of a meaningful, safe relationship. It's a support system for tough times and a cheering section for good times—and a comfortable chair in which to pass the time on any day in between.

Love and Respect

Earlier I spoke of accepting yourself as a hand-crafted, purposefully designed being. Author Neil T. Anderson's workbook *The Steps to Freedom in Christ* addresses, among other things, the problem of low self-image among those who call themselves Christians. His conviction (which I echo) is that if we, who acknowledge ourselves as followers of Jesus Christ, are ever to regain a true and accurate picture of who we are, and who we were created to be, we must agree with what God's Word says about us. Below are some statements of truth from Anderson's powerful self-help material (the emphasis and selection are mine).[4]

In Christ

I am...God's *child* (John 1:12)

I am...Christ's *friend* (John 15:5)

I am...a saint, *a holy one* (Ephesians 1:1)

I am...*complete* in Christ (Colossians 2:10)

I am...*free* from condemnation (Romans 8:1-2)

I am...*confident* that the good work God has begun in me
will be perfected (Philippians 1:6)

I am...*a temple* of God (1 Corinthians 3:16)

I am...God's *co-worker* (2 Corinthians 6:1)

I am...God's *workmanship*, created for good works
(Philippians 4:13)

Don't those words encourage you to love and respect yourself, my brother or sister in Christ?

What if you aren't a Christian? God's Word still has a message for you regarding your high intrinsic value—if you are willing to receive it. In Romans 5:8 the apostle Paul says this:

> God demonstrates his own love for us in this: While we were
> still sinners, Christ died for us.

And in Lamentations 3:22 we read, "Because of the LORD's great love we are not consumed, for his compassions never fail." You see, whether or not you choose to accept it, you are passionately loved and greatly valued. So much so, that rather than allow you to live recklessly apart from Him, God sent his only Son, Jesus, to the cross so your relationship with the heavenly Father could be restored.

This very day you can choose to love and respect yourself simply because God says that you're worthy of being loved and cherished. And it only makes sense that if you cling to your own self-image over what God has said of you, you will *always* have difficulty keeping food in its rightful place. (After all, the God who made you also made food.)

Find a way to love and respect yourself, then the new you can live in harmony with food.

Looking Forward

The "old you" spent an awful lot of time looking backward. That was then, and *this is now.* Although the new you must navigate through today, you must always keep your eyes on your future. You are engaging in this fight against food addiction because it robbed you of your past, made your days miserable, and was promising to steal your future. That thought must stay clearly etched in your mind as you live your life forward.

You no longer need to drag around the chains of food addiction… you can live free. Sure, you have the niggling fear your food addiction will once again rise up and take over. If it does, acknowledge it, confront it, denounce it, and move past it (as we discussed in the last chapter). Fix your eyes on a healthy, joy-filled, productive life! As you've read through the personal stories between the chapters in this book, I hope you've come to the conclusion that victory can indeed be won. May it be for you as it was for them.

The *Rest* of the Story…

The final aspect of your new life I would like to address is your sleeping habits. Even the amount of sleep you get at night affects your appetite! *Is no stone left unturned?* you ask. Sorry, I don't want to stop being 100 percent truthful and thorough…I want to make sure you have every advantage against food addiction.

Some people erroneously believe that the only connection between hunger and fatigue is that if a person feels tired during the day, they'll look to eat more food to energize them or wake them up. Not so. This is certainly a part of how inadequate sleep affects your food intake, but there's an even more compelling scientific reason why you need to get between seven-and-a-half to eight hours sleep each night. During the stages of deep sleep (stages 3 and 4, for those of you who know a bit about sleep cycles), your brain produces two hormones that regulate your appetite. One hormone, *leptin*, suppresses your hunger, while the other hormone, *grehlin*, increases your hunger. When you do not get adequate sleep, your brain produces too much appetite stimulant and not enough appetite suppressant. Armed with that knowledge, aren't you beginning to feel a bit sleepy?

❧

I congratulate you for making it through this book. I prayed about each word I would write, and I have been praying for you, dear reader—that this information would guide you out of the prison of food addiction and into a wonderful new world of health, longevity, and harmony with food. The new you will not be an instantaneous transformation, and I hope that you're not under that impression. Transformation is a journey—but one definitely worth taking! Thank you for allowing me the opportunity to walk this part of your journey alongside you.

Blessings to you, my friend,
Lisa

Resources for Healthy Living

≈◊≈

Making My Story Yours

≈◊≈

Notes

Resources for Healthy Living

Tools

Body mass index (BMI) online calculator:
www.RestoringYourTemple.com.

Books

Arthur Agatston, MD. *The South Beach Diet Super Charged.* New York: Rodale, 2008. Web site: www.SouthBeachDiet.com.

Danna Demetre. *Scale Down: A Realistic Guide to Balancing Body, Soul & Spirit,* updated edition. Grand Rapids, MI: Fleming H. Revell, 2005. Web site: www.dannademetre.com.

Carole Lewis. *First Place 4 Health.* Ventura, CA: Regal, 2008. Web site: www.firstplace4health.com.

Jennifer Rothschild. *Self Talk, Soul Talk.* Eugene, OR: Harvest House Publishers, 2007.

Organizations

First Place 4 Health: www.firstplace4health.com/forums/index.php.

Overeaters Anonymous: www.oa.org/all_about_meetings.htm.

Making My Story Yours

...continued from chapter 6.

In John 17:3, Jesus gives this definition: "This is eternal life: that they may know you, the only true God, and Jesus Christ, whom you have sent." Accepting Jesus as Lord is far more than just "fire insurance"—protection from eternity spent in hell. When you choose to turn your brokenness over to Jesus Christ by admitting your sinfulness and confessing your need of a Savior, three amazing things happen:

1. Your past is forgiven.
2. Your present becomes filled with purpose.
3. Your future (eternity in heaven) is secure.

Does that sound good to you? It did to me! It was everything I longed for.

So how can you make Christ your own story? It is quite simple. God knows your heart and can hear your prayers (even when they are uttered inside your mind). If you are done trying to go through life alone, pray the prayer below with a sincere heart, and you will restore the relationship the God of the universe always intended you to have with Him. I realize you don't feel worthy, and the truth is you're not—none of us are. But that's okay. Salvation is a gift from God, so no one can brag about how they were able to obtain it or how much they deserved it.

Prayer of Salvation

Dear Lord Jesus,
I confess I'm a sinner in need of a Savior.
I thank You for paying the penalty
for my sins by dying on the cross.
I accept Your gift of forgiveness
and eternal life with You in heaven.
By the same power that God used
to resurrect You from the grave,
I declare that my old self has been made new.
I give You full control of my life.
Make me into the person
You created me to be.
All for Your glory!
In Jesus' name,

Amen.

What do you do now? Grab a Bible and learn about the things that make God happy. And then, just as the Nike ads say...*Just do it!*

> Whoever has my commands and obeys them, he is the one who loves me. He who loves me will be loved by my Father, and I too will love him and show myself to him (Jesus, in John 14:21).

Notes

Chapter 1—Putting on the Pounds

1. *American Journal of Clinical Nutrition,* August 12, 2006.

2. "Obesity and the risk of myocardial infarction in 27,000 participants from 52 countries: a case-control study," *The Lancet,* November 5, 2005.

Chapter 2—The High Cost of Overweight

1. R. Klesges, M. Klem, C.L. Hanson, L. Eck, J. Ernst, D. O'Laughlin, A. Garrott, R. Rife, "The effects of applicant's health status and qualifications on simulated hiring decisions," *International Journal of Obesity,* June 14, 1990, 527-535.

2. E. Rothblum, P. Brand, C. Miller, H. Oetjen, "The relationship between obesity, employment discrimination, and employment-related victimization," *Journal of Vocational Behavior,* 1990; 37:251-266; R. Puhl, K.D. Brownell, "Bias, discrimination, and obesity," *Obesity Research,* 2001; 9:788-805; "Fat Execs Get Slimmer Paychecks," *Industry Week,* 1974; 180:21.

3. N. Katz, "Reinventing Mid-Life: Sleep, Aging, and Overeating," Institute for Natural Resources, June 2008.

4. National Cholesterol Education Program (NCEP) Expert Panel on Detection, Evaluation, and Treatment of High Blood Cholesterol in Adults (Adult Treatment Panel III) 2002, "Third Report of the National Cholesterol Education Program (NCEP) Expert Panel on Detection, Evaluation, and Treatment of High Blood Cholesterol in Adults (Adult Treatment Panel III)," final report, circulation 106:3143-3421.

5. Paul S. MacLean, "Exercise-Induced Transcription of the Muscle Glucose Transporter (GLUT 4) Gene," *Biochemical and Biophysical Research Communications,* 2002; 292 (2): 409-414.

6. M. Guerre-Millo, "Adipose tissue hormones," *The Journal of Endocrinology Investigation,* 2002; 25:855-861.

7. National Cholesterol Education Program (NCEP) Expert Panel, circulation 106:3143-3421.

8. E. Calle et al., "Overweight, obesity, and mortality from cancer in a prospectively studied cohort of U.S. adults," *The New England Journal of Medicine,* April 24, 2003; 48 (17):1625-1638.

9. H.K. Yaggi, "Obstructive Sleep Apnea as a Risk Factor for Stroke and Death," *The New England Journal of Medicine,* November 10, 2005; 353:2034-2041.

Chapter 3–Why You Binge

1. N. Katz, "Reinventing Mid-Life: Sleep, Aging, and Overeating," Institute for Natural Resources, June 2008.

2. K. Wandler, "Clinical Management of Eating Disorders and Co-Occurring Substance Abuse," *Christian Counseling Today*, 2008; 16:1:40-43; Katz.

3. D. Aaron and T. Hughes, "Association of Childhood Sexual Abuse with Obesity in a Community Sample of Lesbians," *Obesity*, 2007; 15:1023-1028.

Chapter 4–The Not-So-Merry-Go-Round of Food Addiction

1. David Hawkins, *Breaking Everyday Addictions* (Eugene, OR: Harvest House Publishers, 2008), 14-15.

2. Frank Minirth, Paul Meier, et al., *Love Hunger* (Nashville: Nelson, 1990), 40.

3. John Bradshaw, "Bradshaw on: The Family" (Deerfield Beach, FL: Health Communications, 2008).

4. Minirth et al., 59.

Chapter 5–Stuffing Down Your Emotions with Food

1. Beth Moore, *Stepping Up* (Nashville: Lifeway, 2007), 21.

2. Judith Wallerstein, "The Long-Term Effects of Divorce on Children," *Journal of the American Academy of Child and Adolescent Psychiatry*, 1991.

Chapter 6–Healthy Ways to Purge Your Pain

1. Frank Minirth, Paul Meier, et al., *Love Hunger* (Nashville: Nelson, 1990), 121-134.

2. Minirth et al., 133.

3. *Overeaters Anonymous* (Rio Rancho, NM: Overeaters Anonymous, 2001).

4. Minith et al., 133.

Chapter 8–You Are What You Think

1. Jennifer Rothschild, *Self Talk, Soul Talk* (Eugene, OR: Harvest House Publishers, 2007), 10.

Chapter 9–Best-Laid Plans...Dealing with Setbacks

1. George Ohlschlager, "A Personal Journey with Addiction," *Christian Counseling Today*, 2008; 16:1:8.

2. Frank Minirth, Paul Meier, et al., *Love Hunger* (Nashville: Nelson, 1990), 192, emphasis added.

Chapter 10—Presenting...the New You!

1. James B. Calvert, "The Mystery of the Senses," *Brain and Mind*, ed. Silvia Helena Cardoso, February 23, 2009, www.cerebromente.org.br/n16/mente/senses1.html.

2. B. Wansink, J.E. Painter, J. North, "Bottomless Bowls: Why Visual Cues of Portion Size May Influence Intake," *Obesity Research*, 2005; 13:1:93-100.

3. B. Wansink, K. Van Ittersum, J.E. Painter, "Ice Cream Illusions: Bowls, Spoons, and Self-Served Portion Sizes," *American Journal of Preventive Medicine*, 31:3:240-243.

4. Neil T. Anderson, *The Steps to Freedom in Christ* (Delight, AR: Gospel Light, 2004), 23.

About the Author

Lisa Morrone graduated magna cum laude from the physical therapy program at the State University of New York at Stony Brook in 1989, receiving a Bachelor of Science degree in Physical Therapy. In addition to her college education, Lisa has taken more than 30 continuing education courses in the area of orthopedic physical therapy. As a physical therapist, Lisa has been treating patients in the field of orthopedic rehabilitation for nearly two decades. In 1990 she accepted the position of adjunct professor at Touro College, Bay Shore, New York, which she still holds today.

At Touro College Lisa instructs in both the Entry Level and the Post-Professional Doctorate Programs in Physical Therapy. Presently Lisa co-teaches Musculoskeletal II (Spinal Orthopedics), Kinesiology (the study of bones, muscles, and joints and their roles in the human body), and an advanced elective on Spinal Muscle Energy Techniques (evaluation and treatment specific to the spinal joints). Her past teaching credits also include: Massage, Extremity Joint Mobilization (evaluation and treatment of the joints in the arms and legs), and Spinal Stabilization Training (core strengthening of the trunk, hips, and shoulder-blade muscles).

Lisa's two books, *Overcoming Back and Neck Pain,* and *Overcoming Headaches and Migraines* were published in 2007. Lisa is a graduate of both the speaker and the writer tracks of the She Speaks Conference (Proverbs 31 Ministries), where she was assessed at the highest level of proficiency. As a speaker, Lisa has taught in both secular (community and medical) and church-based settings, and has been interviewed on national TV as well as international radio. She makes her home on Long Island, New York, along with her husband, daughter, and son.

Restoring Your Temple™

Within Christian circles, one's physical body is often referred to as the temple of the Holy Spirit. The reason for this is found in 1 Corinthians 6:19, where the Bible says, "Do you not know that your body is a temple of the Holy Spirit, who is in you, whom you have received from God?" Temples are places where worship takes place. But what exactly is worship? To quote author Rick Warren,

> Worship is far more than praising, singing, and praying to God.
> Worship is a lifestyle of *enjoying* God, *loving* him and *giving* ourselves
> to be used for his purposes. When you use your life for God's glory,
> everything you do can become an act of worship.

Romans 12:1 further tells us to "offer your *bodies* as living sacrifices, holy and pleasing to God—this is your spiritual act of worship." God has plans for your body...physical plans. Your hands and feet are meant to be used as His hands and feet on this earth. So whether He calls you to raise children, teach Sunday school, or work with teenagers or the homeless, you need a physical body that is ready for action. Scripture says, "The harvest is plentiful, but the workers are few." Oftentimes this is because the workers are at a doctor's appointment, going to physical therapy, or are simply so tired they can't get off the couch!

It is the intent of **Restoring Your Temple** to ready the Body of Christ to perform the work of Christ. The longer you live in good physical health, the more you will be able to enjoy the abundant life God has promised to His children.

Visit Lisa Morrone's Web site, **www.RestoringYourTemple.com,** for

- BMI (body mass index) calculator
- downloadable headache charts
- dietary trigger list
- a home exercise program for those suffering with jaw pain (TMD)
- further help with issues of physical health and well-being
- a source of "Lisa-tested," quality health-related products
- quick tips for back, neck, head, or jaw pain
- guidance on how to find a good physical therapist
- Lisa's personal testimony

Achieve Lasting Changes with Other Resources
from Lisa Morrone

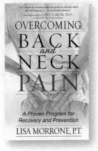

Overcoming Back and Neck Pain

From 20 years of teaching and practicing physical therapy, Lisa Morrone gives you a way to say no to the treadmill of prescriptions, endless treatments, and a limited lifestyle. This straightforward, clinically proven approach offers the most effective exercises, guidelines, and lifestyle adjustments for back and neck problems, showing you how to...

- benefit from good posture and "core stability"
- strengthen and stretch key muscles
- shift to healthy movement patterns
- recover from pain caused by compressed or degenerated discs
- address "inside issues" that affect your body's healing capacity—nutrition, rest, and emotional/spiritual struggles

> *"The treatments Lisa recommends are practical, well described, and well illustrated...An invaluable resource."*
> JOHN LABIAK, MD, ORTHOPAEDIST AND SPINAL SURGEON

Overcoming Headaches and Migraines
Clinically Proven Cure for Chronic Pain

If you're looking for practical help and answers for chronic or debilitating headaches, physical therapist Lisa Morrone has them. Twenty years of teaching, research, and hands-on treatment have given her a thorough, broad-based perspective on head pain. She helps you discover how to...

- uncover the *source* of your head pain and avoid unnecessary medication
- eliminate pain originating from neck problems or muscle tension
- ward off migraines and cluster headaches by pinpointing and avoiding your "triggers"
- find a qualified hands-on practitioner
- get free from negative emotions that can keep you trapped in head pain

A comprehensive resource to help you get back a life you can enjoy and share.

> *"A gift to headache sufferers and those in the health professions who are committed to helping them."*
> —HOWARD MAKOFSKY, PT, DHSc, OCS
> HEAD PAIN EXPERT

More Help with Spiritual-Emotional Issues
from Harvest House

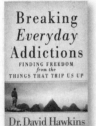

Breaking Everyday Addictions
Finding Freedom from the Things That Trip Us Up
Dr. David Hawkins

You've tried going for a few days without drinking coffee, checking your e-mails, or watching TV, but your good intentions seem to get you only so far. Such repeated behaviors can easily become true addictions that control you and limit your ability to make good choices. *Breaking Everyday Addictions* shows you how God can lead you to freedom. It points you to up-to-date answers for questions like these:

- Is addiction a disease? If it is, are addicts responsible for their behavior?
- Why do anorexics and morbidly obese people continue their self-destructive behavior?
- What is the appeal of gambling against nearly unbeatable odds?

With the information and practical steps Dr. Hawkins provides, you can create a program of recovery that will help you and the people you love regain control and build happier, healthier lives.

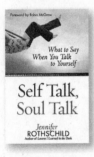

Self Talk, Soul Talk
What to Say When You Talk to Yourself
Jennifer Rothschild

Have you ever noticed the things you silently tell yourself—and believe? *"I could never do that." "They don't like me." "I am such an idiot!"*

Phrases like these endlessly flow through your mind and pool in the depths of your soul. How can you replace these lies with truth? Popular author and Women of Faith speaker Jennifer Rothschild shows how you can stop the flood of negative self-talk and fill your mind with life-giving biblical principles.

Discover what David the psalmist, Deborah the prophet, and other biblical personalities said to themselves, and you'll experience new freedom and vitality as you dive into a refreshing stream of truthful soul-talk.

To learn more about other Harvest House books
or to read sample chapters, log on to our website:

www.harvesthousepublishers.com

HARVEST HOUSE PUBLISHERS

EUGENE, OREGON